Also by Jean Giono

Joy of Man's Desiring
The Song of the World
The Horseman on the Roof
The Straw Man

Blue Boy

Jean Giono

Translated by
Katherine A Clarke

COUNTERPOINT
WASHINGTON, D.C.

Library of Congress Cataloging-in-Publication Data
Giono, Jean, 1895–1970.
[Jean le bleu. English]
Blue boy / Jean Giono ; translated by Katherine A. Clarke.
p. cm.
ISBN 1-582-43051-9 (pb: alk. paper)
I. Clarke, Katherine Allen.   II Title.

PQ2613.I57 J413 2000
843'.912—dc21   99-046034

FIRST PRINTING

Cover Design by Amy Evans McClure

COUNTERPOINT
P.O. Box 65793
Washington, D.C. 20035-5793

Counterpoint is a member of the Perseus Books Group.

10   9   8   7   6   5   4   3   2   1

BLUE BOY

CHAPTER I

MEN of my age here remember the time when the road to Sainte-Tulle was bordered by a serried row of poplars. It is a Lombard custom to plant poplars along the wayside. This road came, with its procession of trees, from the very heart of Piedmont. It straddled Mont Genèvre, it flowed along the Alps, it came all the way with its burden of long creaking carts and its knots of curly-haired countrymen who strode along with their songs and their hussar pantaloons fluttering in the breeze. It came this far but no farther. It came with all its trees, its two-wheeled carts, and its Piedmonteses, as far as the little hill called Toutes-Aures. Here, it looked back. From this point it saw in the hazy distance the misty peak of the Vaucluse, hot and muddy, steaming like cabbage soup. Here it was assailed by the odors of coarse vegetables, fertile land, and the plain. From here, on fine days, could be seen the still pallor of the whitewashed farmhouses and the slow kneeling of the fat peasants in the rows of vegetables. On windy days, the heavy odors of dung heaps surged in waves along with the broken, bloody bodies of storms from the Rhône. At this point the poplars stopped. The carts rolled noisily into the jaws of the wayside inns with their loads of corn flour and black wine. The carters said, "*Pòrca madona.*" They sneezed like mules that have snuffed up pipe smoke, and they stayed on this side of the hill with the poplars and the carts. The chief inn was called Au Territoire de Piémont.

In those days, our country was made up of meadows and fair orchards that used to unfold in a magnificent springtime as soon as the warm weather came up the Durance Valley. They knew how to recognize the approach of the long days. By what means, no one knows. By some bird cry or by that burst of green flame that lights up the hills on April evenings. They would simply begin to flutter while the frost was still on the grass, and, one fine morning, just when the bluish heat weighed upon the rocky bed of the Durance, the gaily flowered orchards would begin to sing in the warm breeze. That we have all seen from the time we were mere urchins in our black school smocks.

I remember my father's workroom. I can never pass by a shoemaker's shop without thinking that my father still exists, somewhere beyond this world, sitting at a spirit table with his blue apron, his shoemaker's knife, his wax-ends, his awls, making shoes of angel leather for some thousand-legged god.

I was able to recognize strange steps on the stairs. I could hear my mother saying below, "It is on the third floor. Go up, you will see the light."

And the voice would reply, "*Grazia, signora.*"

And then the sound of the feet.

They stumbled on that soapstone step near the top of the first flight. The loose boards in the landing rattled beneath the heavy boots. Their hands pressed against the two walls in the darkness.

"Here comes one of them," said my father.

"*Putana!*"

"That is a Romagnol," said my father.

And the man would enter.

I remember that my father always gave them the chair near the window, then he would lift his spectacles. He would begin to speak in Italian to the man who sat erect, hands on thighs, all perfumed with wine and new corduroy. Sometimes it took a long time. At others, the smile came almost at once. My father spoke without gestures, or with very slow ones, because he held a shoe in one hand and the awl in the other. He would talk until he saw the smile. It was useless for the other to haul out papers, to tap on his papers with the back of his hand.

"*Pòrca di Dio!*"

Until the smile appeared my father talked on, and sometimes the other would say in a hushed tone, "*Che bellezza!*"

Then the man would smile.

Moreover, they did not come to my father at once. I do not know by what miracle they came. It must have been transmitted to them, like the knowledge of the swallows, or perhaps marked in some corner of the inn, carved with a knife in the wall. Some sign, a circle and some crosses, a

star, a sun, a mark that must have said in their wretched
language: "Go to Père Jean's."

A sign that could not be seen unless one were lost, lost
like a poor little mouse. A sign that must have been marked
on the weeping wall: the wall that one leaned against to
weep, and then one must have seen the sign carved in the
stone, and he came to Père Jean's.

When I stood near the slope to watch the passage of the
long carts loaded with wine, I saw them come: Romagnols
and Canavezzani. They sang of *dolce amore*. They wore
broad felt hats cocked on one side, their shoulders straight,
and they would stop and stand with their legs spread to
watch the girls go by. Between that moment and the time
they must climb our stairs holding onto the wall on both
sides, there was enough feasting and games of *Mora* to put
their eyes out, and at last their heads would nod and their
fingers grow stiff as iron.

First the smile. Then my father would write letters to
the King of Italy. At that time I had great faith in the letters to the King of Italy. I admired that humble shoemaker's
bench, the penny ink, the penholder with its pen fastened
to the wood by a pig bristle, and then my father's hand all
marred by black scratches turning clumsily as it wrote
"Sire."

Now I know, Father, that it was you who performed the
miracles.

"Go up, you will see the light."
That evening we were just about to go down. It was

high time for supper. My father had already picked up the copper lamp.

"Wait," he said.

Someone was singing on the stairs and the step was sure and swift: a step that could see in the dark by prescience, that knew the solidity of things.

"I wonder who it could be," said my father.

The other came toward us through the night, along the walls and the echoing shadows of our hall and the religious mystery of our ancient convent dwelling. He was singing.

"Who can it be?"

He was a handsome man, young and blond. He filled the whole doorway. A great dark blue woolen beret, pulled down into a point above his brow, made a heart-shaped aureole about his head.

"Torino?" said my father.

"Turin, yes," said the other in French with just a twang of accent. "Commune of San Benedetto."

He began to talk at once. The recourse of the smile was not for this one. He himself was smiling all over. He was one big smile. At the same time he had such easy gestures, such a well-oiled movement of his body, such a skilful waving of his long lean fingers, he was so sure of himself, handsome, young, and fair, that he cast a spell by the very grace of his radiant vitality.

"*Christou*," he said, "perhaps I am the sickest one. I was told to come and see you. Is it here?"

"Yes, this is the place," said my father.

The man looked around the poor dingy workroom with

its litter of leather scraps and the great chandeliers of spider webs hanging from the ceiling.

"Explain if you are in a hurry, otherwise come back tomorrow. You see, we were just about to go down to supper."

"I saw that," said the man. "The table is set downstairs, but the missus told me to come up. Eh, yes, it is urgent."

"Well?"

"The women. They love me too much."

My father set the copper lamp down on the corner of the sewing machine. He took out his tobacco pouch and filled his little white clay pipe.

My father had the time to fill and smoke three pipe-fuls. It is true that they were little Gambier pipes of the Aristophanes brand, the bowl no bigger than a young girl's thimble. I watched him smoking, not with his usual calm, but like a pump he drew in and puffed out the smoke without stopping. Beneath his heavy brows his eyes grew darker. Two or three times he said, "And then, and then, quick."

He released the blond young man from his glance only to take the tobacco from his pouch.

I understood little of what the man was saying. It flowed from him like a plaintive song, like the whining of a dog hungry for a caress. Some of the words fell upon me like stones into a still pond. I was all stirred with shimmering circles which made my heart flutter as they widened or broke suddenly in my throat in little waves of cold, bitter water. For me it had only the force of a song, but all the force of a song. He was transfigured by it, he, the speaker, as if anointed with a light of richer oil than the pale gleam of our copper lamp. As from bursting seeds, I heard new villages blossom about me and live, with their streams of carts, of plows, of torrents, of sheep, their flocks of chickens and flights of swallows and crows. Mountains swelled beneath our floor, lifting me high up into the heavens as on the swell of some giant sea. And I stood up there, a poor ecstatic shipwrecked creature, torn from my father, snatched from the good solid haven of his mouth and from the beautiful bird-haunted foliage of his beard, from the soft hill of his cheek. I stood there aloft in the spray of the high wave, alone, naked, bruised, rubbed by some bitter salt until the blood flowed, but fronting a vast new country, the arena of all the winds, rains, and frosts, and the great blue cyclone of liberty billowed before me amidst banners of swirling sand.

My father took his pipe from his mouth.

"Poor devil," he said.

He said that to this blond-haired man who all at once seemed broken and dead as if someone had fumbled among his vitals with both hands and had withdrawn the little mechanism that had caused the fingers and tongue to move in such a fine seductive way.

My father sat a moment looking at the man who was now still and mute.

"Your name?"

"Djouan."

He picked up the lamp.

"Come and eat soup with us."

We went downstairs, I following my father who was

carrying the lamp. Behind me Djouan's foot was groping for the steps. He stumbled. He saved himself by catching hold of my shoulder.

"*Pardoun, bòccia*," I could hear him whisper humbly.

My mother made her usual grimaces and shruggings behind the cupboard door. As for me, I had already taken the plate from the sink board.

"Put him there," said my father, "opposite the mirror. Take off your beret," he said to him. "Make yourself at home. This is the soup of poor folks that you are about to eat."

We had sausage soup. My mother asked Djouan if he preferred the potatoes mashed or whole. He had turned away and was slicking back his hair with the palm of his hand.

"Pauline," said my father, "do you remember when you passed through Chorges?"

"No," my mother replied.

"That time you went to Remollon with the little one?"

"I was sick in the coach. I did not see anything."

"This man has come from Chorges," said my father, "and he has been up to some devilment there."

I remembered that roadside village. A gypsy camp, a stone camping ground, a traveler's halt. The days and nights filled with the squeaking of axles, creaking of wheels, cracking of whips, the rumbling of stagecoaches, shouts, calls. The heavy odor of the stables foamed in the wake of the loaded carts as they set out from the inn. The waiters stood waving lanterns. A girl ran after a tilbury.

The coach for Gap was starting off, its roof piled so high that it caught in the branches of the plane trees. The horses coming from Italy sensed the halt and neighed as they wound around the mountain road. I remember our arrival as night was falling. It was cold. The icy air came in through the cracks of the windows. The postilion was stamping his feet to warm himself. The horses steamed in the lamplight as if they had emerged from boiling water. Under the wheels the road rang hard. I saw my mother, pale and moaning, her lips without a trace of color, and her head knocking against the side of the coach. Outside, nothing but a valley of barren schist, a twisting green mountain stream, the night and the wind. And then all at once our windows were filled with the hearty laughter of an inn with its door wide open and lighted to the back of its throat. A man in a sheepskin coat was smoking his pipe in front of the door. The coach stopped. It smelled of the hearth, the plate, and the lamp.

"In Chorges itself?" asked my father.

"No," said Djouan, "on a farm."

"In which direction?"

"La Menestre."

"What were you doing there?"

"Oh. . . ." That meant: as a matter of fact, I wasn't doing anything there, it was just chance.

"I had stopped with a bad foot," said Djouan.

"The wife or the daughter?" said my father.

"The wife."

"Let him eat," said my mother.

"He can eat and talk at the same time," said my father. His chin beneath his beard was hard. He added, "The man up there must find it hard to eat, too."

"I don't give a damn for the man," said Djouan.

"Or that you have destroyed his rest and his appetite?"

"I don't give a damn for that either."

"Or that you have taken what belonged to him alone?"

"The woman doesn't love him any more. She loves me. She suits me fine. She is young. Everybody's free."

"That's not what I am talking about."

"You should also think," said my mother. . . .

"I am talking about his peace," said my father.

Djouan had taken out his great mountaineer's knife, broad at the handle like a sickle and finer at the tip than a pigsticker.

"What do you mean, his peace?"

"I know those farms up there," said my father. "You know them, don't you?"

"Yes, it's just the same at Suza."

"Exactly. To live in a place like that you have to have peace."

"That's nothing to me."

"Yes, it is," said my father.

"I tell you it's nothing to me," said Djouan.

"What's that you've got around your neck?"

My father pointed to Djouan's neck and I saw a red string.

"*La Madònna.*"

He drew forth a cloth scapular decorated with an orange-colored bleeding heart.

"I said peace," said my father.

The soup was eaten.

"It was his aid and his help," my father continued. "A man is like a rubber ball. At times, to make himself rise, something has to strike against him. He cannot do it by himself. If he is deserted, he takes two or three hops in the grass and he stays there dead. See?"

With his hand he imitated the bouncing of a ball. He went on:

"He has the woman, what you left of her for him, what he does not know. You have the medal."

"I'd like us to be even," said Djouan.

He cut the string with his knife. He laid the cloth heart on the table.

"I'll leave this with you."

After a moment he added, "Is that all right, boss?"

He kept his hand over the bleeding heart. He said "boss" to my father who was nobody's boss, not even his own. His lips were trembling and his eyes as big as one who has just seen the approach of Death.

"A little better," said my father. "It is fairer that way."

Djouan slowly withdrew his hand. He stood up and put on his beret.

"*Compagnie!*" he said, raising his left hand in salute.

He opened the door and went out, leaving it wide. Outside a steady rain was falling.

CHAPTER II

I WENT to school to the Sisters of the Presentation. It was usually my mother's girls who took me. Sometimes Antonine, sometimes Louisa, sometimes another Louisa.

Antonine was redhaired and abrupt. Her firm hand jerked my wrist. She took long steps. She laughed as she eyed the boys and then her narrow lips could be seen opening over sparkling teeth as though they had been split with a knife. At times her glance was gathered in one corner of her eye as if she had let all that purple viscosity of her ordinary glance run into the corner in order to spurt it from there into the boys' eyes as from the spout of an oil cruet. I saw that very distinctly. After each glance I was afraid I'd find blank orbits and see the boys go running off with the color of Antonine's eyes. One might be afraid of anything, for, upon leaving me at the wrought-iron gate of the school, she had the same glance for me, and I know very well that all the rest of the day shimmered with purple crescent moons, and that I could look at nothing else, flowers, box hedge, nor the statue of the Virgin, without its being surrounded by a dancing and shining swarm of those constellations.

The first Louisa was smooth, sweet, and white like a sugar almond. Before setting out she would look into the little mirror, smooth her hair, straighten her lace collar, get out her little powder box.

"Yes, yes, Louisa," my mother would say, "you look very well, my dear."

Louisa's little hands were warm and fluttering like birds. Every time a horse galloped past, or at every street cry, she drew me so close to her that my head touched her thigh. And each time I was astonished to feel beneath her skirts something big, warm, and moving. Could it be that under those skirts—always clean, beautifully made, fresh and flower-strewn like a hawthorn hedge—could it be that they were filled with some naked, purring creature?

Louisa's eyes were clear and round and always looked one straight in the face with the innocence of childhood that had persisted through its loveliness, and because of it. She faced the wind and the street teeming with horses, porters, wheelbarrows, and men carrying planks of wood: she faced it all with her sugar-almond cheeks and her beautiful quiet eyes. Would you dare? she seemed to be saying. This little child and me, *me?* This *me* was so sweet, so smooth, so white! I buried my little hands in her warm ones. I looked up at her: she smiled back at me. We walked in step, I straining a little to attain the smooth, slow rhythm of her high-heeled stride, and sometimes she hummed a little song all scented with her fragrance which bore us along as on a cloud.

A cloud!

It was a cloud that must have inhabited her skirts and not that warm creature I had never seen, that I would have loved to see, very much—at any rate without much fear—and which rustled softly beneath innocent Louisa. At the gate she would bend down and kiss me, and I would go into the school licking my lips.

Louisa the Second did not often come. She was not sorry. Neither was I. She never talked. She worked. She never raised her eyes. She worked. She would escort me quickly. She longed to get back to her work. She was from the country. Her father owned a big farm. She boarded with us and was learning ironing in my mother's establishment, not so much to make a trade of it as to acquire the skill of the accomplished housewife. Her loud colors, her big hands, her great common sense, her firm step, all were objects of laughter in the laundry. Her peasant solidity was plain to see. She carried her purse in a cloth pocket that hung beneath her dress, and when she entered a shop for a purchase, she sought a corner where she could lift her skirt. With her it was a silent walk in which I felt I was being dragged along. She put into it all the stiffness necessary to make me feel that she was the mistress, but at the same time she showed for the fine little boy that was I all the pliancy he required.

Fine little boy! I mean as to clothes, because for the rest I had a long, thin, unattractive face redeemed only by tender eyes. But in what a majestic starched collar were my shoulders encased and by how many hands was the magnificent sky-blue silk of my tie puffed and bowed before handing me over to Louisa the Second. They knew that she could not be counted upon if some part of my costume should come undone on the way and they delivered me into her good rough hands only when I was completely ready and shining. We would set out. From below when I looked up, I could only tell that Louisa the Second's eyes were green, judging by the light that was watching, from under her downcast lids, the place where we both set our feet. She held no mystery for me. I was not afraid of losing her when I left her at the gate: I knew I should find her there in the evening, always the same, and she would say before letting me go, "If you have to go to the toilet, say so."

She was the only one who used the formal *vous* in speaking to me.

I saw her a year or so ago. . . .

In fact, I have seen all three of them in the last few years, and I said, "Antonine!"

Then: "You were a darned old rascal all the same! Do you remember when you put me in the clothes basket that Sunday I had on my new suit, and when you made me fall into the brook?"

"Don't speak of it," she said; "your mother must still shudder when she thinks of it."

I have met Louisa the First's husband and have shaken hands with her big boy, and have listened to all three of them as they talked. I thought that in my heart I had always been slightly in love with her. She is just the same, not changed a bit.

But Louisa the Second: in spite of myself I said, "Mademoiselle Louisa."

She is left all alone, the mistress of her farm. One feels that she is hard and bitter, straining with all her might toward a goal that is not a woman's goal. And now she looks you straight in the face, too directly, with pleading hot eyes.

The garden of our school was like a big fruit full of pulp and juice. The walls that pressed it about made it spurt and bubble; lilacs ran over on all sides; the great boxwood spattered the walls of our little classroom with shadows and odors, and the ivy seething with bees foamed like jam froth over the high terrace wall. The paths were paved with little inset pebbles. Sister Dorothée was the paver. She could always be found crouched in a bubble of shade. She would lay her little stones in arcs of a circle of which the width of the path showed only a segment: the visible and peaceful segment sheltered by the convent. The rest of the circle went trailing off into the garden, into the world beyond, far, far away, beyond the walls and hills that were barely visible, and God alone knows where it traveled before returning once more to the hands of Sister Dorothée.

We were not long in discovering that this was a punishment task and one had to have sinned in order to plant the little colored stones. It was always Sister Dorothée. She was not much more intelligent than we. We used to go crawling along on all fours behind the boxwood in search of her. Presently we would come face to face.

"Where are you going?" she would whisper.

"We've come to see you."

"Hide."

We would hide.

"Who is in charge of the yard?" she would ask.

"Sister Philomène."

"Then there are at least five punished already."

"Six."

"And you four will be, too, for coming to see me. That will make?"

"Ten! Can we help you?"

"No. It amuses me."

"Would you like some chocolate?"

"Who has some?"

"Me."

She would wipe her hands on the under side of her robe. "Come," she would say.

There was a hiding place under a great rose laurel. It had so much fragrance, such a strong odor, that merely getting under it was intoxicating. This fragrance pressed upon my eyes. In no time at all everything I saw was deformed. The faces of my little playmates melted in the blue shadow like a lighted candle, melted and ran, leaving spots in the grass, and there were spots dancing in the shade like bits of melted suet floating there, bearing an eye, a mouth, an ear, or the little shiny red window of a cheek. Sister Dorothée would stretch out on the grass. She became a black world humped with mountains and hills, hollowed

with dry and silent valleys, waterless, treeless, quite deserted, and as if despised. All that was alive was the happy
region of her face where her mouth was eating chocolate, where her lips finally made a moist sound, where beneath a slanting ray of sunshine her cheek grew velvety
with a blond down that seemed, in my intoxication from
the fragrance, to undulate and wave like a vast sea of ripened grass.

We would stay there hardly breathing. Yonder, the yard
paved with large tiles rang under racing feet and games.
The walls crackled with shouts like a sputtering frying pan.
One could hear the sound of the iron rings, of the horizontal bars, and the ropes of the trapeze creaking on their
hooks. In the little classroom three culprits were spelling
out the lesson in a monotone.

The laurel was really as big and strong as a man.

"Sh!" said Sister Dorothée.

We held our breath.

There was the sound of crunching gravel. Keys rattled.
A willow wand was softly tapping against a robe with
nervous little twitchings like a cat that lashes itself with
its tail as it looks about. Sister Philomène! She touched the
abandoned paving with her foot. She was searching about
her with all her cunning: her ferret's nose was sniffing
the air, her sharp eyes piercing the shadows. But the laurel
was really as big and strong as a man. One felt well
sheltered beneath it. It was all thickness and brave deceit.
One loved it so much for that, that one trusted it completely. Sister Philomène sighed. She gave one more look
at the arcs of the paving: the arcs of circles that went curv-

ing out into the world beyond the hills. She sighed, yes, several times, and vanished almost noiselessly, like a big cat, with only the sound of the wand nervously tapping her robe.

They generally laid my friend Paul flat on the table in front of the raised seats. Sister Clémentine chased the tiny children away with her long arms that made the sound of flapping wings.

"Clear the table quickly: the inkwells, the copybooks. There, that slate, quick."

Meanwhile, Paul was mopping his nose with his handkerchief which was red with blood. He waited quietly, separated from the world by his bleeding, touched by God, the indolent object of Sister Clémentine's solicitude and everyone's curiosity. As soon as the table was cleared, they laid him flat upon it, his head back, after saying to him, "Paul, let your nose alone."

Sister Clémentine and Louisa the First are for all eternity straight and fair in my heart like lilies.

What fascinated me about Sister Clémentine was the middle of her body. At rest, there was nothing, so to speak, but the thick, coarse rope girdle and the folds of her black fustian, as I remember it, three broad folds that lay like garlands over her breast and ten folds that descended to her feet. She wore her robe rather short, showing her ankles. Standing motionless, her arms bent to hold her book, her head erect, she had the nobility of a column. But—

But, sometimes in our morning class, when, withdrawn from the noisy world of the street and the town, we could hear the convent quiet flowing in upon us with its cooing of pigeons and the brushing of the lilacs against the walls, Sister Clémentine would begin to walk. At this moment as I write, here with my strong cigarette in the corner of my mouth, my eyes smarting, my lighted lamp, and the night in the valley pressing against the window with its phosphorescent trails of peasants' carts, I have just put down my pen to think over all my experiences as a man. Certainly, to the secret eyes of my senses, there has come the dance of almost every seductive serpent in the world.

I have never experienced a joy more pure, more musical, more complete, more surely born of equilibrium than the joy of watching Sister Clémentine walk.

It began like the rising of a curving wind. The boards of the platform uttered a magnetic little cry. She was walking. She wore felt sandals, the soles of her feet made a gentle padding sound. Along the column rose an undulation that recalled waves, the neck of a swan, a moan. It was so ample and so firm, it came so directly from the depths of the earth that if the undulation had mounted to Sister Clémentine's neck it would have broken it like an iris stem. But she received it on the fine springs of her hips, she transformed it into the rolling of an outbound ship, and the whole upper part of her body, breast, shoulders, neck, head, and cornet, shuddered as when a sail swells to a puff of wind.

Stretched out on the table, Paul was bleeding without touching his nose. He was as still and pale as a corpse. The blood formed a great clot on his nostril. Then it stopped flowing. Paul blew hard and the loosened clot slid down his cheek like a little flower at the end of a shining stem of fresh blood. The blood-stained handkerchiefs had been spread over the back of a chair by the window. It was like a slaughtering of the innocents. Presently the lay sister rapped and entered with her odor of herbs and onions.

"He's been stuffing that thief-weed up his nose again," she said. "You are a fine sight, Monsieur Paul!"

Sister Clémentine picked up the invalid. He lay limply in her arms. He looked up at her with big ox eyes. Down in his throat he was mumbling some indistinct plaint.

"Yes, my sweet," she would say as she wiped his face.

She moistened a corner of her handkerchief with her saliva and wiped Paul's blood-stained mouth with the tips of her fingers.

"Take him away," she said to the converse. "Go along, my dear."

And she ran her hands through his hair.

There were only two or three of us who knew that for love of Sister Clémentine, for the hand run through his hair, for that saliva on his lips, Paul snuffed up thief-weed. He had dried enough of it to fill an old shoe polish tin. There it lay hidden like a treasure beneath our feet. One had only to raise slightly the board in the platform. There was enough of it to make us all bleed like bulls.

My first intercourse with a virgin took place before people assembled, one Easter Monday, in a flowering almond orchard. I mean my first importance intercourse.

The convent school was, as is proper, sustained morally, pecuniarily, and beautifically by everybody that walked in silk in the town. The notary's wife, the pharmacist's wife, the retired commandant's lady, the wife of the beadle, the wife of the landed proprietor, of the justice of the peace, of the clerk, the Children of Mary, the harpists, all the young ladies made of sugar, Delphine, Clara, the troop with downcast eyes and hands encased in mittens, all who were corseted in whalebone, all who walked like a flock of herons, belonged to the convent group. They nourished, polished, shined the convent like a good creature who dispensed glory and moist tongue lickings.

It was surprising that my father should have consented to hand me over to that school. At the time of the decision it had simply been a question of daily bread. My father was old. He worked by himself. If he worked well and alone in his high, dark room in the back of the house, without a shop, without a display window, with only his trade, he was a slave to the town. A pair of shoes cost twenty francs. When he made them they were strong, and, he used to say, one was sure of walking on leather. But at that time, in order to be sure of walking on leather, one had to belong to the upper crust. The proposition had been put to him cleverly.

"This fine child," the lady, who had come into the workroom holding her nose and had seated herself on an imponderable part of the chair, had said, "this fine, delicate child who looks so much like his mother! You are not unaware, Monsieur Jean, that before she married you, Mademoiselle Pauline was a member of our congregation and I dare say was so zealous that we had all conceived great hopes for her. She married, she made her choice. We have never wished to influence anyone, and we know that you are good to her in spite of the difference of religion."

My father stopped her with a wave of his hand.

"There is no difference, Madame."

"They say," she went on, "that you are a Protestant."

"I would be," said my father, "I admit it without the least shame, but I must tell you that I am not. What might have led you to believe it is that I read the Bible and that I discuss it. In reality, I am not anything. I believe in God, and if I differ with my wife's belief, it is only that she believes that God has created branch offices on the earth, with bureaucrats and employees who dispense tickets to His kingdom, and I have imagined Him as being great enough to do all that by Himself, and moreover, that when one has need of Him, He is to be found everywhere."

The lady tossed her head and the ostrich plume in her hat made its shadow dance on the wall like a marionette.

"We know," she said, "you are a very good man just the same, and it isn't out of perversity . . . Pauline has told us that you let her go to Mass. . . ."

"She is free," said my father.

"Remember," said the lady, "that we have been very nice to you, too. For Pauline's sake you have been given the resoling of the convent, my husband has ordered his hunting boots of you, and I know that Madame de—

would like to see you about an old man in the poorhouse
in whom she is interested and who will have to have his
shoes mended before long."

"Well," said my father, "what is it that you want?"

"Look," she said, "you know that we have a school at
Saint Charles. You are intelligent enough to know that
there is no comparison between the education and instruc-
tion that the good sisters give and what the teachers in the
public schools teach, aren't you? The children are kept
until six o'clock. There are gardens. The cost is twenty
sous a week. . . ."

"Pauline is free," said my father.

There followed a silence in which nothing could be
heard save the creaking of the leather sole that my father
was sewing.

The lady took her leave. I lighted her down the stairs.
She went down to my mother.

My father had said: "If he is of my blood, he will make
his own decision. Send him, if it gives you any pleasure."

On Easter Monday there were special vespers in the
little church of Saint Charles. There were no stained-glass
windows but honest water-green glass, a little on the bottle-
green shade, and through these windows could be seen
the top of the horizontal bars with ten swinging ropes
bearing rings, the trapeze, and the swing. The altar was of
gilded wood crowned with great stars. The sacristy was
just behind the altar, a simple shelf and a little cupboard.
The priest dressed there: his arm and shoulder were visible
when he was putting on the chasuble.

Early in the afternoon the ladies began to arrive. The hall of the school was filled with greetings. The cold tiles of the parquetry gleamed like lovely black water and the ceramic flowers floated upon them as on a fair, quiet, sheltered pool.

This time it was my mother and my godmother who took me to school. My collar was whiter and stiffer than ever and my tie so blue that my usually blue eyes were that day like little balls of ashes. They had put knitted gloves on my hands, they had threaded the tops of my socks with cunning elastic, and were dragging me toward the school by both arms. My mother dragged me along by one, and my godmother pulled me along by the other. I walked between them like a little captive monkey.

I was to recite the homage to the Virgin.

There was no need to tell me to keep it a secret at home or to tell me not to speak of it to my father. It was enough for me to be near a mystery to become at once the personification of infant silence. Everything that touched the other world I felt I loved intimately like one's native land, like a country where I once had lived and loved dearly and from which I was exiled, but which was still living within me with its weaving roads, its great rivers lying flat over the land like trees with long branches, and the swelling undulations of the shaggy hills whose every track I knew. I felt that I knew all this much better than grown persons, and I knew such games of darkness before which Antonine and the two Louisas would have fled, but which I contemplated boldly with merely a little icy tingling at the tips of my buttocks. I drew from it a sort of superior pride. If Jesus, the Virgin, and even God the Father, had appeared before me, if they had made me their earthly companion, I should not have cried out like Joan of Arc nor Bernadette. The world would have continued in ignorance of it. It would have appeared quite natural to me.

However, what did seem supernatural to me, as impossible to understand as the geography of invisible lands through which the immense flock of the gods streamed in clouds of dust, was, to my mind, the existence of these women who were buzzing about in the convent hall. That they should be endowed with a body and speech, that was supernatural. From them came sounds of glass beads, bracelets, rustling silk, and sputterings like the sea breaking on the shore. What connection could there be between them and the Virgin to whom I was about to talk? And even what connection could there be between them and little Sister Dorothée, still undergoing punishment, and who had just passed by with her hands full of little round stones?

Two little boys and two little girls carrying banners made a square around me. They looked at me out of the corner of their eyes and terror palpitated in their glance like a great fly. Sister Dorothée looked at me, too, before disappearing through the half open kitchen door.

"Farewell, farewell!" she seemed to be saying.

The ship that was to bear me toward the mystery was taking shape about me under the direction of great unseen forces. I no longer had any little playmates or friends. They were now only planks in the ship. They piled about me and fused together to transport me, and their lighted

tapers were golden nails that danced like the pegs of sailing vessels when the sea and the wind begin to sweep along
their sides.

Only the ship owners and the shareholders were calm.
The Mother Superior was arranging the procession. She
straightened a flag, bent a taper forward, tapped a cheek
with her finger, smiled at young Catherine de Faidherbe
and even knelt in front of her to smooth a flounce of the
beautiful white moiré dress. Of all things! After all, *I* am
the chief, I thought. *I* am the important one in all this. Who
is to do the talking when we arrive yonder? Who will step
first onto the solitary shore, before the Virgin? Who is to
receive the great divine gaze? In short, who is to be the
victim? Me. Very well. Then, wouldn't it be wiser to
take me a little aloof from the crowd, to place me behind a
coil of rope or a keg of pitch, and there, in quiet, to make
the friendly gestures that give a person courage? Wouldn't
it be wiser to do that than to pet that silly old Catherine
de Faidherbe who was there only in the capacity of banner
at the stern?

"Stand still," whispered my mother.

The garden gate was opened.

The sun and the springtime were struggling outside with
gusts of warm wind. The almond blossoms were flying in
all directions.

A clap of the hand and the ship of children slipped into
the sea.

> "To our tender Mother
> Bring our wounded hearts. . . ."

The organ was bellowing lustily. *My* heart was not wounded. It was all stroked, caressed, expanded, as if it were floating on the sea beside the ship. The motion, the cadence of the steps, that ship's wind that had struck us on the starboard, blowing all our tapers at once—all the children had cried: "Ah! Ah!" like the birds in May—everything burst into song upon our fine launching. We were in the garden, far inside. Surely I recognized the familiar scene: the boxwood, the great fig tree, the rose laurels, but through the open windows the choir leader was singing at the organ:

> "To our tender Mother
> Bring our wounded hearts. . . ."

The banners flapped their wings like great doves. Torches of burning lavender were passed from row to row behind me and I could hear, running through the trees, the Virgin's fat servants who must be calling to her, "Madame, Madame, here they come!"

We were coming.

The Virgin dwelt in the midst of the almond orchard. Everything was in bloom and the grass was green. It was a lovely house. For pillars it had the black tree trunks that looked like sick men casting their twisted arms to the sky. For a roof, a great mass of flowers. The carpet was that thick curly salad green, dandelions that spurted juice under one's tread.

As always, the Virgin was on her pedestal. She was made of sandstone riddled with holes by the rains, and I knew that under ordinary circumstances . . . under ordinary circumstances this is what she did. One evening I had approached her. The wind was blowing as usual. A fitful wind, sometimes cold as water and at others it warmed your cheeks as before a brazier. The Virgin of soft stone was all worn by the rain. The wind was making her sing.

Today, she was silent. There were too many people. *I* knew her. I felt that she was not as she usually was, that this was not the day, that we had chosen the wrong time; that if she had had time she would have had her maid say to us that she was indisposed, as my godmother sometimes did.

The best thing to do would be to tiptoe away, to go, to close the doors and windows, to hush the organ and let her recover in her house of trees, under the caresses of the sun and the flowers.

I was not in command, I who knew her. And it was of no concern to those who had paid for the expedition. There I was alone before her.

The others stood in silence behind me, waiting.

The Mother Superior looked at me.

"Begin, my child," she said.

I raised my eyes to the Virgin.

"Good Mother," I said, "you who are the fair open pomegranate and the ripe orange. . . ."

Suddenly I burst into sobs.

"She is dead! She is dead!" I cried.

It was fairly easy for me to escape when everybody rushed forward. I only caught a glimpse of my mother to whom the matter was being rather coldly explained.

I found Sister Dorothée in the hydrangea walk.

"You are not going to crawl on the ground in your fine suit," she said to me.

"Yes, I am," I said.

She did not dare to contradict me and preceded me on hands and knees under the laurel.

She kissed me.

I gave her some chocolate.

"Sister Dorothée," I said, "Sister Dorothée, the Virgin, you know, the Virgin?"

"Yes," said Sister Dorothée, "the Virgin, what about her?"

"She is dead," I said.

"Oh, yes," said Sister Dorothée.

I saw that she had known it for a long time. She laughed as she ate her chocolate.

CHAPTER III

ONE EVENING my father had just shut the street door when someone knocked. There came two very hasty, heavy raps and a strange voice called pitifully, "Père Jean!"

"What is it?" said my mother, pale as a reed.

"We'll see."

My father lifted the iron latch. Outside, the man was stamping on the sidewalk with his heavy boots. My father held the door slightly open. I shall never forget that lost hand. It was black and greasy. It had pushed in from the street. It was pressing against the door to open it wide. It was distracted and plaintive like a rat that is being chased with a club. The door opened. The man thrust himself into our house and shut the door.

"Lock it, lock it," he said trembling, and he pointed to the bolt.

My father pushed the bolt.

There we stood, the three of us, inside the door: my father, myself, and the man. A little farther away, behind the table, my mother was lifting the lamp and now we could see that the newcomer was thin, ragged, and his face was blue beneath his beard.

He had just heard the bolt slide home. He said as if to excuse himself, "Coupard. Monsieur Coupard."

"Did he send you?" said my father.

"No, but he spoke to me."

"Where are you from?"

"I was working at Salon when they arrested me."

"And then?"

"The gendarmes took me to Digne. I wanted to urinate. They untied my hands. I struck. I ran."

"Far?"

"To the edge of the town."

"Quiet," said my father.

There was the sound of people running down the street. They passed close by the door. They turned to the left into the street that leads to the dark quarters.

"Pauline," said my father, "make some coffee. Have you eaten?"

"No."

"Give him some bread and cheese."

I went over and stood by my mother.

"Your father, your father," she mumbled, shaking her head.

She looked at them. They were both seated yonder in silence. The man was slowly getting his breath.

A room was arranged for him upstairs on the third floor, near my father's workroom, in the storeroom where the olives were kept. Before going up, the man had said, "I'd like to wash my hands."

A mattress was laid on the floor.

"Sleep and don't worry," said my father.

The man extended a hand that was now like a fair, tranquil pigeon. "Thanks, comrade."

Before going out of the room, I turned. The man had taken a little mirror and comb from his pocket and he was combing his beard.

Our house was a dual one. It had two voices and two faces. On the first floor was my mother's laundry establishment. A huge table padded with a white cloth. My mother would sing like a bird: "Cherry-time," "The Golden Wheat," "Griefs Are Mad Things," "Black Stockings," "Frou-frou." Louisa the First harmonized. Antonine whistled like a man. Louisa the Second nodded her head to keep time. There were also two little apprentices who went with enormous baskets to deliver the laundry. They were taking Madame Pangon's dress from the line.

"Look out for the loops!"

They laid it in the basket. They piled up the handkerchiefs. They folded the panties.

"The lace outside."

"For what it signifies," said Antonine.

"Be careful, the little one is here."

"He'll find it out for himself."

"Come here and let me kiss you, my sweet almond."

They would take my face in their warm, moist hands, scented with the ironing.

The butcher's wife and the baker's wife, who lived next door to each other, came to spend a few moments.

"I don't know what I have here on my thigh, it's the size of a hazel nut. Feel."

They would lift their skirts. My mother would feel. Antonine would feel, the Louisas, the apprentices.

The town crier came in with his bugle under his arm.

"Play a tune," demanded Antonine.

"Silly," scolded my mother.

The crier stood there impudently, twirling his arms, and jostled the linen hanging on the lines.

"Ah! Good heavens! Mademoiselle Delphine's caps!"

Antonine's beau passed by the window.

"There he is again," she would say. "I am going to empty a bucket on him like a dog."

"We'll have to throw it on you too," said my mother. "Watch what you're doing; you are going to get scorched, you little slut."

A door opened onto a corridor. From there the street could still be heard rubbing against the shop, but a few steps more and one entered into another world. The face of the house here was shadow and silence. You went down one step and you were in the inside court. In broad daylight during the winter the night stayed there from morning till evening. In the summer, toward noon, a drop of sunlight slipped into the court like a wasp and then flew off.

I came home from school at four o'clock. I was now a pupil at the shabby little *collège* which the town had banished beyond its wall up on the threshing floors toward the hills.

It was nice in my mother's laundry. They sang. An-

tonine smelled of plums, Louisa the First of vanilla. Louisa
the Second munched hard candies.

"Go keep your father company," my mother would say.

In the courtyard, at that hour, it was always dark. In the
sausage shop next door a machine ground pork meat without respite. You could hear the purring and hiccuping
sound through the wall. The stairs were broad and of easy
ascent. Our landlady said that one could ride up them on
horseback to the second floor. She would say that with her
hands clasped and with her eyes wide and round beneath
her cap.

In addition to the song of the meat grinder that seeped
through the walls, you could hear large rats running over
the tiles, and then if you stood still for a moment, the sound
of a big stone falling deep down into water below. It was
the ancient well that was speaking. Its door had been locked
and it had been left to rot within. The well digger had
said that down inside were two races of creatures: white
toads, completely white, without eyes, and as big as
plates. They swelled up like bladders in order to float.
"They stay that way, year on end," he had said, "never
stirring. They grow old, floating there without air and
without light; floating on that water that is thicker than
oil. Toads, yes, and snakes, too. Skinless snakes, or with a
skin as thin as cigarette paper, just enough to hold their
heart and vitals together."

I would climb the stairs, and each time my foot touched
the soapstone step in the darkness, I was afraid I was going
to touch one of those white toads that might have escaped,

or slip, as on a ripe apricot, upon a snake's warm heart.

The man who had entered our house that evening had never left it. For two weeks his meals were carried upstairs to him.

He was there now, on the other side of the workbench, his elbows on his thighs, his head bent forward full in the light of the copper lamp. He was rolling a cigarette.

"No," my father was saying, "you have not a revolutionary spirit, you have the spirit of justice, that is all."

"You have read Bakunin?" said the man.

My father nodded his head toward the great iron-bound trunk that took up a whole corner of the room.

"I have him in there."

"Jean Grave?"

"He's there, too."

"Laurent Tailhade?"

"Yes."

"Proudhon?"

"Yes."

"Blanqui?"

"I knew him at Puget-Théniers."

"I was a member of the Society of the Seasons," said the man.

"That is no longer in existence," said my father.

The man pushed all his hair back with the palm of his hand. I could see his hand plainly now. It had become human and good. One felt that it was no longer alone in its fear for its life and its groping search for a friendly touch, but that it was once more attached to a man's body by a good arm. It was long and slender, it gave the impression of being skilful and of good will. The fingers were thin and agile. Around the nails, in the grooves of the skin, the white ring peculiar to plasterers was still visible. When the man spoke he held his open hand out in the light, palm up, with its fingers flexed and the broad palm hollow, bare, and scarred with labor.

"It has been reorganized," he said. "Proudhon, good. If you only know one man you cannot believe Proudhon. Here, inside of me . . ."

He struck his breast with his fist. His closed fist was like the head of a hammer.

"Here, inside of me, there are only two desires and pleasures. Here, inside of me, there is only that mechanism that sends us in search of prey for our mouths or our . . ."

He glanced at me.

"And for our . . . You understand? To help others, that is not inside me. Mutuality? Hell! All that does is to perpetuate little private property. So. They have reorganized Blanqui's Society. I belonged to it, see?"

He extended his hand into the light. It was spread wide. As he spoke, he slowly closed his fingers as if he would grasp the whole light of the lamp.

"Battle. Yes. There is nothing but that for us. That is all that is left."

I was no longer conscious of him. I saw only his fist held out toward us, as big as a world.

"I have already told you," said my father. "You have the spirit of justice, that is all."

One morning the man came down to get some hot water from my mother's stove. He asked, "Haven't you a pair of scissors?"

He went back up to his room with his bowl of hot water and Louisa the Second's little embroidery scissors.

He cut off his beard. He left a tiny patch at the tip of his chin. He turned up the ends of his moustache. I was there while he was doing it. He looked over at me as he twisted his whiskers between two fingers.

"It's hard to make them stay up," he said. "They have never been used to it."

In fact, as soon as he let go of his moustache, the ends gently dropped and then the man reappeared. He reappeared as he had been with his full beard, as he had been that evening when he had burst into our house. You could recognize him at once. It brought back his sad look. I believe that he finally waxed the ends of his moustache with a bit of pitch.

When evening came, I was unbuttoning my blouse to go to bed when my father said to me, "Stay here, we are going out."

"You are going to take the boy?" asked my mother in astonishment.

"That will allay suspicion," he said. "It will merely be a walk."

Upstairs in the attic, the man was ready. He had made a fine round belly that filled his vest. My father looked him up and down.

"What do you think of it?" asked the man.

"Yes," said my father, "that is bourgeois. That will do

for this evening. But day after tomorrow you'll have to think up something else. That belly will bother you. From here to Switzerland, it is a good many kilometers."

We went out. The street was deserted. It was eleven o'clock at night, toward the end of autumn. The weather was soft, even slightly disagreeable. The night air sweated a bitter little dew.

We immediately left the main street and entered the dark by-streets that were called "beneath the bells." A maze of little streets twisted in a net about the church, just beneath the campanile. It seethed like the veins in an ash leaf: it was blacker than the night, it smelled of stink and the stable. There were odors of bread and dried fagots. The dull sounds of stamping could be heard behind the walls. A small window bled great globs of light that splotched the pools of liquid dung.

"The oven," said my father. "They are making the bread."

He added: "And you, are you getting accustomed to the air?"

"Yes," said the man, "I am used to it, don't fear."

He was listening to the sounds of work.

"You might think they were fighting in there."

We turned into the little street where the stables were. The horses were snorting and pawing the ground. Goats were pulling at their chains. Lambs were calling for their mothers' udders. A cat seated in the shadow looked at us with eyes like two little glowing red stars. There was only our step in the town. We passed through the peasant quarter. On the paved street was the mud of the plains;

the dirt from the hills was drying in great clods. A heap
of gorse fagots was shriveling against the wall. It already
smelled of fungus. At a stable door the chopped-up trunk
of a fig tree had been dumped. A donkey brayed. A dog
watched us go by. The sound of his collar could be heard
as he raised his head. Strings of garlic rustled beneath the
little projecting roofs over the doors. There was a light at
only one window on the ground floor. I looked in as we
passed. A woman was standing beside a bed, stirring a bowl
of herb tea with a spoon.

There was only our step in the town. We were going
toward the boulevards, toward the country, toward the
trees. The man's step was as firm as my father's long
stride.

"Listen," he said stopping short, "a fountain!"

It was beating drum taps in its basin.

Suddenly we came out onto the boulevard. We had an
unobstructed vision of all the glowing coals of stars and
we could hear the hills moaning beneath the hand of the
wind.

"Comrade! Comrade!" said the man.

He had seized my father's arm, and I was aware that his
hand was trembling. Liberty!

"You are crying," said my father.

"When they arrested me," the man said, "I was building
a mantelpiece in a new house. It was a fireplace that would
draw like the devil. Never any smoke, if the wind was
from the north or south, never; it was my secret. On the
front of the mantelpiece I had drawn two oak branches
with my thumb."

I could see his thumb move across the starlight. It was thick and black like the root of a tree.

"Three months in prison at Salon. It opened onto a corridor. It was there that I tore off my shirt. They took me to Avignon in a box loaded on a cart. Five months in Avignon. And this is the first time, since. . . ."

The town slept behind us like a dead hive. From time to time a rumbling came from it as if its store of honey were settling deep in its cells. All was sleeping. The town breathed only in its fountains. The clock struck midnight.

The world was now speaking above men with its voice of wind and stars.

"Comrade," said the man, "it will be like the day of the Last Judgment, do you hear?"

We had stopped under an elm. The silent little owls could be heard flying through the foliage.

"*We* shall be the ones who are to be the final judges of evil and injustices. The wretched will come out of the ground, and all the earth will be split in crevasses. In the fields, in the meadows, in the hills and the mountains, in the middle of the hardest roads, the earth will be heard cracking, it will be seen breaking up into stars, rising like the mouth of a mole hole, and the wretched will spring up about us like plants. You, comrade; I, comrade; this little fellow."

His hand rested on my head as if to mold dreams within it.

"The workers and the peasants, we are now wrapped in our shrouds and they have tied the bands tight about us; and have wound the band around the chin as for the dead to prevent us from speaking. It will be like the Last Judgment; when the trumpet sounds the shrouds will fall from our shoulders, our mouths will be unsealed. I can't describe it, I can see it."

"I see," said my father.

"The first time I saw it," the man said, "I was building in an olive grove. I had made the four walls and the ceiling. I was on my knees in a corner, with my trowel in my hand; I was spreading plaster on the white walls. Around me, nothing but the smell of plaster. For some time I had been feeling something in my head like a bird that was awakening. All at once I was drunk with it. It seemed to me that a great form with colored wings was struggling in the doorway to get to me to announce. . . . From that moment, I saw. They can put me in prison; they can put me where they will. I bear the revolution.

"Comrade, we, the proletariat, workers and peasants, we have solid fists, we shall shake the heavenly chestnut tree and the stars will fall to the earth with all their burrs."

"That will cause bloodshed," said my father.

"Stink."

"I'd rather be a healer," said my father. "You must put me where I can heal."

"There won't be any hospital, comrade; there won't be any wounded after the Judgment. It will be a second Flood."

He stood a moment breathing in the night.

"Farewell," he said.

"What?" said my father.

"I must be off. Now. I have just made up my mind as I listened to the sounds about me."

"This evening?"

"This evening."

"We had planned for the day after tomorrow. It is far from here to Switzerland. You'll have to have food. You'll have to have some money."

"Give me what you have on you."

I heard my father fumbling in his pockets.

"Thirty-five sous. Jean, have you any sous?"

I felt in my pocket.

"Four sous, Papa."

"This is all we have. If you would come back, we would prepare your sack."

"Liberty," said the man. "Liberty. No friends, no chains, no gratitude. As naked as Adam."

He said no more. Then I heard him walking rapidly away on the soft ground.

CHAPTER IV

A
S SOON as it grew dark I used to go and sit beside
my father's workbench. He would light his
tall copper lamp. Then he would take down
the cages.

He had five cages filled with birds: canaries, chaffinches,
goldfinches, and a little cage for decoy birds in which he
kept a solitary nightingale. The nightingale's cage had a
putrid odor. He had to be fed on earthworms chopped into
bits. My father cut the worms with an iron fork whose five
prongs he had sharpened with his three-cornered file. He
also fed his nightingale flies. He would catch the flies in his
hand, then give them to the bird. The nightingale stuck
his bill through the bars to pierce the fly's abdomen. A
drop of blood, thick and white like pus, oozed out. When
the fly was a big one, or if it was a May beetle, my father
would cut the insect in half. First he gave him the thorax
with its blue wings.

"The poorer bit first," he said.

Then he would offer the little honey-filled sack of the
abdomen.

46

The lamp lighted and regulated, my father would take down the cages. He put them beside the workbench so that the birds would be in the rosy light of the lamp, and after a time they would all begin to sing.

I would listen especially to the chaffinches and bullfinches. In order to persuade the nightingale, he had to be slightly in the shadow, near the pail where the leather was put to soak. Then he would begin with little sobs.

"Listen, listen," said my father.

All the birds grew silent. Huddled together on the little wooden perches, they sat there fluffed out and scared, the transparent tips of their feathers trembling.

"Listen."

The nightingale was softly weeping to himself. A slender little voice tinted gray and red with pain.

"Listen, he's going to begin."

And then I realized that there was to be a change. The odor of the rotten food rose in two or three great bubbles and immediately the terrible rolling song of the bird burst forth.

I sat at my father's left, in front of the big cupboard. On that side, our house adjoined the wall of the house next door. It was a cracked and rickety hive, gaping with fissures and zigzag apertures, in which rooms were rented by the night to the vagabonds of the poplar-bordered road. Like my father's workroom, these rooms had windows only on the court in which sheep were lodged. They came from up in the mountains. They bleated for a day or so. Then they were still. I used to watch them. They would stretch their necks out on the black straw and remain thus with no sign of life save their breathing. On Saturday a butcher would come and open the door. He would arouse the sheep with kicks. The creatures stood up; their bellies were black with dung, and they would go limping away.

Sometimes the head of a man or a woman would appear at the windows next door. The women immediately looked up toward the light and that shred of pure sky that covered the top of the court like a flat stone. The men spread their arms on the windowsill; they bent their heads and stared at the sheep, silent, motionless, save for their breathing.

As the house next door faced on two sides of the court, I was able to obtain a better view of the people who lived in the rooms nearly opposite my father's workroom. There was a little girl over there. Her father went to the cafés with a card-table mat. He would spread the mat on the floor, in the sawdust, roll up his shirt sleeves, clap his hands together, give a leap, and there he was standing on his hands and walking with his arms as if they were his legs. Sometimes he would return to the mat, slowly bend his arms, touch the mat with his chin, and then right himself with an air of profound satisfaction. He would take a saucer at random from a table and pass it around. The little girl was much younger than I; she was four, I think. I had seen her when she first came over there. She wore a red dress and a huge yellow bow in her hair that was stiff and black like an iron helmet. At first, like all the women, she had looked up at the sky, but soon she bent her head over the sheep below.

She would call to the sheep, holding out her little hand

to them and snapping her thumb over her closed fingers.

"Come, chicky; come, chicky," she would sing with trills like those of our nightingale.

The sheep paid no attention.

One evening, as the nightingale had just finished his song and was picking in his meat bowl, I heard people coming up the stairs next door. They were newcomers. They were going to live next to us, separated from us only by the wall. A chest with nails on the bottom was being scraped noisily across the floor. I heard the door shut and then two men began to speak. They talked on and on without a pause, one endless word like respiration. My father was listening, too. He tapped on the bullfinches' cage.

"Sing," he said.

The birds sang. The talking ceased. After a moment the birds began to eat at their seed. The men could be heard talking in low tones like a purring.

My father tapped his finger on the chaffinches' cage. "Go on!"

The chaffinches burst into song but soon stopped, for chaffinches do not like the lamplight.

The nightingale shook his iron manger and sang. My father listened without venturing to stir his hand that held the cobbler's knife nor his legs that were clasping the beaked anvil. The song was like tiny sparkling red moons and in the midst of them a great dreary sun whose rays of white knives turned dizzily as it thrashed through the night.

When the nightingale had ceased its song, my father laid down his cobbler's knife. He picked up the lamp and said to me, "Come, let's go down."

There was not a sound to be heard.

My father longed for a little garden. His desire blazed in our midst like a fire. We were both burned and warmed by it. As soon as he had finished eating at noon, the song of the wind in the street drew my father. He went out to walk along the paths in the outskirts of the town. He must have examined every enclosure and even measured the land by pacing with his long stride from one corner of the wall to the other, and then he must have calculated how much money it would cost at so much a meter. He profited by these walks to bring back food for the nightingale. In the meantime, I went to our high staircase and I climbed up to meet the sun. Above my father's workroom was a vast attic, sonorous as the hold of a ship. A broad window, looking down into the sheep court, permitted one to see, over the roofs, far away, the sparkling of the river, the sleepy hills, and the clouds swimming like fish with their bellies dark with shadow. It was impossible to live in the lower stories of our house without dreaming. There was too much decay on the walls, too much darkness that smelled of mushrooms, too many sounds in the thick walls. One had peace only on leaving this house, and in order to escape, one could use the sounds, the shadows, the strange faces that the dampness had traced on the walls. One could use the broad window.

I can still see the marine depth that murmured beyond

the town. The whole valley steamed beneath the foam of the roads. The twisted spray swept up from freshly harrowed fields. The wind went on its way and all trembled in its wake. You felt that it was moving steadily forward, that even while it was here, its eyes were gazing upon new lands outspread and wheeling before it like great multicolored birds. You felt that it was both strong and gentle, that it sufficed you to lean firmly against its flank to be borne away into the wide world. You felt that it sowed this longing within you like a wild deliberate seed and that later you would be rent by enormous roots that stirred like the tentacles of an octopus. I felt the wind take root in me. Now, when I have to try to heal within myself those outbursts of bleeding and sharp pain within my being, I think of those seeds with which I was sown as I stood before the broad window and I always find deep in the wound the little violet serpent.

The moisture rose in the walls to the attic. On the side facing the north slept a gray shadow, crossed sometimes, even in the broad daylight, by the pale flash of a rat. I used often to look at this wall. First I had to let my eyes grow accustomed to it. I could feel my gaze enter deeper and deeper into the shadow. It was like passing through layer after layer of sky before reaching the country. Gradually I reached a point where the darkness grew less dense, a sort of aurora rose along the north wall, and I saw "the lady." It was a splotch of mildew. Her face was oval and slightly rounded. She was green, but the greenest part was in her eyes and all the color of her skin could be only a reflection, the luminous glow, of her gaze. At the place where her mouth was, the disease of the wall had eaten to the bricks, and it was blood-red like real flesh. She was autocratic and harsh at times with herself and me. Those green eyes and that mouth that I coveted, she could hide at will, deep in the mildewed shade. She stayed there all alone although she knew very well that everyone would have loved her had she revealed herself. She directed all my thoughts as she fixed me with her gaze.

Indeed, the emotion of her glance passed from me through my mind in spurts that I alone controlled, speeding toward the wind or toward the mystery of the thick walls, but, as I stood contemplating her, it was she who cast the stone into the still pool of my being. She could be suddenly and magnificently generous; certain of my terrible longings she soothed in herself. At other times she would refuse me the simplest kindness and I would go away trembling, with nothing fixed or solid in my breast. I spent long days of suffering. She never softened at my suffering, but awaited the good season in my heart. When that right moment had come, she awoke in me, with a single look, the song of all my violets and caused the thick jasmine to flower and dance over my heart in the place where the flames dance over the painted heart of Jesus.

This face on the wall had still other powers and charms. It was humanly lovely and sad. Its beauty came from its profound humanity. The brow, the cheeks, the mouth, the eyes, the deep fold that curved on one side of the lips of brick, the hair—all was of defenseless, living flesh, freely offered to the great molding thumb of life, fearless of joys and of griefs. Often, in spite of the implacable hardness of the plaster thought that whitened her brow, I felt in my innocent soil the stirring of the plant of manhood. I felt that it would be sweet later on to accompany and protect this face, to live with it, seek in it consolation for my trials; I prayed with all my secret forces that it might not be only a mildew stain on the stone and I longed so hard for it to become flesh that after a very long time of silence and waiting a living form seemed to touch my dazzled eyes.

Yet, everything around me conspired to prevent me from ever forgetting that face. Unknown to me, secret forces thrust the silent shuttle through the threads. Several days after the installation of the new lodgers in the big house next door, my father went off in search of his garden and I climbed up to the attic to wait for him.

I was looking at the lady. It had rained all night long, a sort of mad rain slanted by the mountain wind, and the north wall was soaked. A tiny drop of water hung in each of the green eyes.

I do not know whether it began with a beginning that could be marked. It must have been alive in the hidden background; its birth was no more than a surging of all earthly matter like a wave rising from the sea.

I heard the sound of a flute.

It seemed to me that the brick mouth was speaking.

It was a sadly gay air. The execution of the flutist was of an implacable rectitude. One felt that his music, before leaving him, had lain coiled like a serpent for a long time in his head. Beside the flute walked a somber violin. They were climbing together up a long ascending road. They had the slow step of those who are going a great distance.

My heart began to take the same long steps that I was to hear ringing in me much later. I put out my hand in the darkness and the lady of the wall put her hand in mine.

At last I came down to my father's workroom. He was already there. The clock in the belfry struck four.

My father was sitting stone still. The birds were as if dead.

"Did you hear the music?" he asked me.

"Yes."

"Your eyes are red."

"I've been rubbing them."

"Your hands are dirty."

"I touched the wall."

"Where have you been?"

"Up there."

Until suppertime we sat in silence. My father had not taken down the cages. He was pulling the wax-end gently and knotting his sewing with two twists of his wrists instead of one so as not to make a sound. The silence whirled around us like sand in the wind. From time to time there was the faint sound of an awakened chaffinch as it tapped with its beak against the manger. A sheep sighed. The night outside seemed to stir with its wings, then lie still sheltering the world beneath its sable plumes. I was motionless, I scarcely ventured to breathe, my gaze passed through the paper lampshade, the walls, the ceilings, until it reached the sweet repose of a glorious countenance of green and red.

Of the two men who played music, one was called Décidément and the other Madame-la-Reine.

One day when I was playing on the sidewalk in front of our house, the former passed close by me. He smelled of over-ripe apple and old leather. I had just time, as my glance mounted the length of him, to see his flowered linen trousers and a pale face from which dripped the two long soft ends of his moustache. I had not heard him coming. He was wearing espadrilles. A little farther down the street in front of the butcher shop he met the fat abbé of Saint-Sauveur. He looked him square in the face and then, at the top of his voice, he cried, "Quack! Quack!" Deliberately he continued on his way, without haste, with his whiskers swaying.

Madame-la-Reine had parti-colored hair carefully brushed and shining. I met him once at the tobacco shop. He said, "Give me a penny cigar."

He was the tallest and the thinnest man that I have ever seen. If he moved a finger it crackled; when he walked his legs and arms crackled, and as he took the cigar his hand made the sound of the crackling of burning wood. He lit his cigar at the lighter and stood there puffing the smoke very fast with his eyes closed.

At table, my father looked at me, then turned his piece of bread around two or three times in his fingers.

"Would you like to learn music?" he asked.

For me, music was full of mystery, and if my father had said, "You are going to learn sorcery," my throat would not have been more taut with fear.

"I don't know," I said, not recognizing my own voice.

And all the warmth of my body had suddenly descended to my shoes.

"I think you are right, you don't know," said my father after a moment's silence. "But that doesn't matter. Just go next door and listen to the men."

"Twenty sous a week," he added for the benefit of my mother who held the purse strings.

Décidément opened the door to me and stood there examining me, his head bent, his eye vacant, while his moustaches gently wept to his vest pocket.

"Here is the little monsieur," he said at last.

Madame-la-Reine, who was fumbling in the big chest, stood up crackling like a piece of kindling and he came toward me.

"Come in!" he said.

He put his hand over his heart.

When the door was closed we all three stood looking at each other. Madame-la-Reine cracked his fingers as he rubbed them together swiftly and his elbows flew out on each side of him like the stumps of wings. Décidément shook his head from time to time, making his whiskers flap. I examined the big dark room, so vast and so high that the daylight reached the middle of it like a little block of ice. At first the walls and ceiling were invisible. It was only after a moment that I was able to distinguish the muscular body of the house about me.

"I think that it is going to be all right," said Madame-la-Reine. "If the little monsieur will be so kind as to come inside. It isn't coming in to stand here and look at each other. Here is something to sit on."

With his foot he drew forward a carpet upon which I sat down. Madame-la-Reine sat cross-legged beside me. Décidément moved back into the shadow.

"I am very well pleased," said Madame-la-Reine. "It is not a question of do-re-mi. Why learn it? What good is it? The fact is, who learns it? Where does it come from? Mystery."

He cracked his long finger as he extended it into the shadow from which Décidément was emerging with his violin and the flute.

Madame-la-Reine took the flute and I noticed that now his fingers made no sound. He bent his head along the wooden shaft, his hands perched on the flute like birds. He looked at me.

His eyes grew dim.

"This is going to be *Monsieur* Mozart," he said.

And they began.

It was dark.

It had been *Monsieur* Rameau, *Monsieur* Scarlatti, and little Johann Christian. We had had *Monsieur* Haydn just as daylight faded. It had lasted until the darkness was complete. Now there was nothing around me but music. I no longer saw the paper that was hanging off the walls, the two mattresses on the floor, the pitcher, the two plates also on the floor, and the big wooden chest. All was dark. Sometimes, in a silence, when they had finished playing, one

of these gentlemen, Madame-la-Reine, would shake his
flute, making it hiss like a horse whip.

"What does the little monsieur think of it?" asked
Décidément.

"Strike a light," said Madame-la-Reine, "we'll see."

He lit a bit of candle.

Then he put the light close to my face.

He began to whistle between his teeth as he saw my eyes.

Turning toward Décidément he nodded his head several
times. Then he stood up and I was conscious that they
were both looking at me in silence.

I say nothing more of my father or my mother. Nothing
existed save the music.

Once my father asked me, "Is everything all right,
sonny?"

He added, "And now, don't you want to learn music?"

"Oh, no!" I said. "No!"

And I began to blush; then I stroked his big hand that
was all scratched and blackened.

On Saturday I took my twenty sous.

"On the chest," Madame-la-Reine told me.

I placed my coin on the chest.

Décidément was peeling potatoes.

"*Monsieur* Mozart," said Madame-la-Reine, "was a little
boy."

"But he was *Monsieur* Mozart," said Décidément.

"Yes," approved Madame-la-Reine.

"*Monsieur* Haydn," he continued, "was an old gentleman. He ate pheasant and drank champagne in a big glass
as tall as this. People lent him chateaux, ponds, trees, and

whole forests of white lilacs. Only, he knew how to forget."

"Yes," said Décidément, "he never let himself be influenced by his digestion."

"And besides," said Madame-la-Reine, "his hand was very supple."

And with his cracking hand he made the gesture of a pigeon's wing that said: "Farewell, farewell!"

"Only," said Décidément, "he understood friendship."

"How are the potatoes getting on?" asked Madame-la-Reine. "Do you want me to help you?"

"No, it's all right," said Décidément.

I touched Madame-la-Reine's arm: "The other day you played something. It was pretty—"

"What?" asked Madame-la-Reine.

"I don't know."

"When?" asked Décidément.

"I hadn't been here yet."

"Where were you?"

"In our attic."

"Were we both playing?"

"Yes."

"What were you doing in the attic?"

I said that there was a green and red lady on the wall up there. And suddenly, from what came into my mind, of her beauty, her compassion, the vast kingdom that she ruled in my heart, it all came back to me.

"This is what you were playing."

I began to whistle the sadly gay air of the flute; I was as one who does not speak with his own voice and with his own head but who is only the instrument of all the hidden forces. The very body of my lady passed between my lips, and the shreds of my torn and happy heart, and the magnificent unfulfilled promises of the great mildew eyes.

Madame-la-Reine stood up. "Bach," he said, "Johann Sebastian!"

Décidément had stopped peeling the potatoes.

"How can you expect," said Madame-la-Reine after a moment, "how can you expect me to guess? He said that it was pretty."

He looked at me: "That is not pretty, Monsieur, it is beautiful."

"Suite in E minor, Polonaise," announced Décidément.

He laid down his knife, picked up his violin, polished it with his coat sleeve. He examined his bow. Gently he touched the strings. Madame-la-Reine wiped his flute with the palm of his hand, he manipulated the free keys. He exercised his fingers in the air, fingers which already, at the mention of music, had become silent as smoke. He put his lips to the flute and softly said, "All right!"

"*Ah!*" sang the flute, "*it was written that for us life would be an old hag.*

"*An old hag with a dripping nose, scaly eyes, and a mouth like a disease.*

"*And she would not be able to stop loving us with her bony carcass and forcing our mouth with her tongue that stinks like an old rabbit skin.*"

"*That is how it is,*" said the violin, "*that is how it is, old fellow, what can you expect?*

"That is how it was written by God. And besides, one can scarcely do otherwise than caress our lover, holding our nose and closing our eyes."

"She shall have nothing but our skin and our blood," said the flute. *"The stench passes into my nose, but I breathe it out through my mouth; it does not remain.* She *only remains in my head, the pure and somber beloved."*

And thereupon, while the violin scolded in low tones: *"Good, you are right, let us go, forward, onward, softly, onward,"* the flute rose, and like a serpent erect in the grass with the joy or the wrath of its flesh, it described the form of that disdainful happiness which inhabits the free mind of pariahs.

As a matter of fact, neither the violin nor the flute said to me all that I have just written, the second time that I heard the Polonaise. I was a little boy filled with the lady in green. But since then I have whistled the air thousands of times, and each time I have recalled the haughty, disgusted faces of Décidément and Madame-la-Reine.

"Bach," said Décidément.

"Bach's *little* voice," added Madame-la-Reine, shaking his flute.

"Jules," said Décidément, putting his hand on the flutist's shoulder, "Jules, do you recall the ascent of the Toccata, and then when you are up there you set your foot in blank despair?"

"Yes," sighed Madame-la-Reine, "the thing is to be strong enough then to do somersaults on your own, without support and without fear for your head. Everything is in that."

"You know that the scoundrels gave him three hundred francs. You can see him, up there, with the thick lips and flat nose of men who had hard-breasted nurses. You can see him up there at the organ during the recessional. This is what he plays. Down below Madame, the butcher's wife, greets Madame, the Prefect's wife; Madame Prefect greets Madame Influential Elector, and the curé counts the collection. 'This business is taking a long time,' he says, 'everybody has gone. Well, Monsieur Bach, let's go to dinner!' "

"I think we have forgotten the little monsieur," sighed Madame-la-Reine in his sad, polite voice.

They both crouched down on the carpet beside me.

"Bach," said Madame-la-Reine looking at me, "was a big gentleman. He ate quantities of soup. That is why he had two wives and twenty-one children. So."

"That explains more than one would think," added Décidément.

"But," said Madame-la-Reine, "it seems to me that a while ago the little monsieur whistled whole measures. He has understood the thread of the story."

"That is what we'll teach him," said Décidément.

From that day, Madame-la-Reine received me each time by rubbing his electric hands together and saying, "Now to work."

They played to me Bach, *Monsieur* Haydn, *Monsieur* Mozart. Afterward, I recited what I had seen.

They would listen to me, approving or correcting.

"No, at that moment, the black swan dips his head three

times into the water then raises it, and each time the little drops of water trickle over his feathers: tralala, tralalalala; each time exactly the same. But we continue to hear the sound of the pond lapping in the grass, and then suddenly the swan lifts up his head and calls. Then the stag—"

"The bassoon," put in Décidément, raising his forefinger.

"Then the stag, as I was saying, emerges from the forest. He has leaves in his antlers and he is laughing like . . . like Monsieur Décidément."

"There," approved Madame-la-Reine. "Tomorrow you shall whistle that for us."

One day Décidément was feeling indisposed and I returned at once to my father's workroom. He was not seated on his stool. He had opened the big cupboard and was standing with his ear against the wall, listening.

"You are back?" he said. "I was waiting for you to begin." And he closed the cupboard.

"You will catch lice from those men," said Antonine.

"Heavens! If he did!" my mother almost screamed.

"I'm only teasing," said Antonine.

While they sat around resting and waiting for the irons to heat, Antonine drew me between her knees.

"Here, let me look."

She began to rumple my hair.

"One," she said, snapping her nails.

My mother rushed forward with quivering nostrils.

"No, it's only a joke," said Antonine. "You get upset over nothing. Besides, if you don't have any it is because you aren't healthy."

"Let me look," said my mother.

And she began to inspect my head from one end to the other.

"Because I, the music, you see, is very lovely. . . . Oh, no, he hasn't any."

Since the arrival of Décidément and Madame-la-Reine, the sheep court had changed.

Behind the fourth window lived a fat woman, without age or color. The window was in a corner where the sun could not reach. The window ledge was all moss-eaten. The woman's sink emptied through a lead pipe bearded with that species of fern that grows on the borders of wells. In spreading, the plant struck against the dirty water and sent out long, skinny, pale stems toward the sparkling stream of the sun. The woman never opened the window. Behind the panes the shadow was the color of water in river bottoms. Only at certain times in midsummer, when even the sheep court smelled of dry dust and the heat of the hills, the pallid face of the woman came and pressed its nose against the glass. In the glaucous dimness of the room swam a white form. It was like a dreary fish. It would come to the window joints to sniff the heavy summer odor. There was just time to glimpse two great eyes without eyebrows and the monotonous swaying head with sagging cheeks, and then with a supple movement it would recede and suddenly disappear completely. The woman had come to live there upon leaving prison. Before that, she had kept a carrier's inn at the junction of the Reillanne and Gambois roads. Only heavy carts passed that way. They say that one night she had gotten into a fight and had killed a man. Her house had caught fire.

Next to her lodged an artisan tanner. He tanned the skins of little animals in his room; skins of badgers, martens, foxes, weasels. In order to dry them, he would hang them on the shutters of his window. There they were, stretched on little stick crosses, and at the slightest wind they would begin to hum and try to fly away like kites. I loved to watch the stretched skins and listen to them. Once, in one of those strong autumn winds that shake the whole town and make the hollow houses moan, two skins, those of a marten and a weasel, flew clean away. They sailed over the roof tops and were never seen again. The tanner went in search of them. He could be heard walking on the roof tiles. All the inhabitants of the sheep court were at the windows, except the colorless fat woman who never approached the glass. They called to him:

"You're going to break your neck."

"Look over toward La Choise's attic, the wind blew that way."

"You are going to break the tiles with your feet and then the rain will come in the houses."

He went off in the swell of the roofs, a tiny figure between the waves.

They called from one window to another:

"He is sure-footed."

"That costs a lot, a marten skin."

"That will teach him to let that stink in our faces."

He came back. He had found only one skin.

The acrobat's little girl also took great pleasure in listening to the skins: the dull buzzing, almost an animal sound, with something of the cry of the dead creature. A great deal of pleasure in watching them, with their leaps and bounds, as if the stripped animals were alive and naked yonder in the hills, standing in the savory awaiting the return of their skins. The little girl was always dressed in red. She would flatten her shoulders and her folded arms on the windowsill, and her yellow and black head seemed to be floating in blood.

In the other rooms were a ditch digger named Tonino, then a couple who had come back from Mexico; the man was from these parts, the woman from beyond the sea. She could be heard singing tuneless songs that were sad and hard to bear because they drew tears to your eyes as pitch draws out splinters from deep in the wounded flesh. She would accompany herself by strumming on the bottom of a pan with her hard fingers.

Besides these, there was, at the lower windows, a Spanish couple, vegetable vendors, with five children. Beneath their room, a little stable sheltered their horse. It was an Arabian horse, with a long mane and a beautiful tail, but so thin that it seemed made of two balls, the head and the crupper joined by a pencil. When it was kept in the stable it would eat its door. It could be heard tearing off the wooden splinters and chewing them with a little trembling whinny that clattered like the wind in the palm trees.

Of the two remaining rooms, one sheltered a mysterious dark man who had been a friar of the Christian order; and the other a young girl, in whose room there was a light every night and the sound of arguing. Every morning, the young girl would open her window, take a towel that was drying outside, and with bucketfuls of water she carefully bathed. She was almost always naked. You could see to her knees.

Yes, the face of this court had changed. In the heart of its misery was born a fine enthusiasm, and in spite of its bad teeth and ugly mouth, it wore through the days an ecstatic smile and an air of joy. It was as though it had a secret love, and was self-sufficient.

One afternoon, the acrobat's window opened. For some time the little girl had not been seen. Décidément and Madame-la-Reine must have been out giving music lessons.

"Hey, you men!" shouted the acrobat. "Music, please!"

I approached the window and watched without being seen.

He had kept on his acrobat sweater under his coat. He was thin and blue with a growth of old beard. His eyes burned in his face.

"Music, I tell you!" he cried again. "It is for the little girl."

Above could be heard the Mexican woman strumming softly.

"Music, in the name of God!" cried the acrobat.

The dark man opened his window. The girl next door to him also. They were listening. Some sheep began to cough.

"Music! Music!"

Then I began to whistle softly. My father said to me, "Go close to the window."

First I whistled that Polonaise of Bach which came involuntarily to my lips just by seeing in my mind the gaze and the mouth of my lady. Then I whistled a minuet by Haydn and a minuet of Mozart.

"More, more!" commanded the man opposite when I stopped to moisten my lips.

I whistled the beginning of a passacaglia and the soft runs of a Scarlatti which had no end but was renewed in its short phrases.

"Enough!" said the man.

And he shut his window.

I heard the girl saying in a low voice to the dark man, "No, it is the cobbler's little boy."

That evening we were told that the acrobat's little girl had died and was to be buried the next day.

"We must go to the funeral," said my father.

He dressed me himself in my Sunday clothes. He wore his starched shirt and Louisa the First tied his black tie for him.

I carried a bouquet of flowers.

My playmates made fun of me, but the young girl of our court looked at me after that whenever she met me in the street.

One Saturday evening Madame-la-Reine said to me, "Tomorrow let the little monsieur fix himself up. We are going to take him to the Spanish grandee's house."

As soon as I got back inside my mother's laundry I told all the workers about it.

"What's that?" said my mother.

"On Sunday," said Antonine, "they are going to Madame Burle's; I heard them."

"Ah, well," said my mother.

She seemed rather flattered.

"And what are *you* going to do there?" she said.

"I'm going to listen."

"If you had learned how to play an instrument, you would play. You see, with your head. . . . And his father, with his ideas. . . ."

"Tomorrow you will see the idiot," Antonine told me.

They dressed me all up, and about three o'clock in the afternoon I went off with the two men.

It was a white Sunday in midwinter, with a great solitary wind. The street was deserted. A dog was howling to the sad sound of the bells. When we reached the town hall square, we turned to the right. We came to a great house corseted with iron gratings. The men rang the bell. We entered. They did not speak and I could hear my big reddish brown tie singing "sh, sh" under my chin.

The corridor was like a chasm and pitch dark. It echoed beneath our step, and the sound was repeated from echo to echo. It vanished all around us in the darkness.

Madame-la-Reine took my hand. His hand was firm and reassuring. It helped me to find the first step and the railing.

Décidément rapped at a door.

"Come in!" came a harsh voice from inside.

It was a large room in which sputtered two three-candled candelabra placed far apart beneath pier glasses of plaster representing cupids entwined with garlands of laurel. The middle of the room was dark and explored by spurts of a tiny squinting hearth fire, stuttering and half stifled by ashes. However, it was this hearth fire that showed me, in the midst of the shadow, a fat, heavy woman, sunk in an armchair and perfectly motionless. The commands came from her.

"Come in! Shut the door! Poke the fire!"

Madame-la-Reine shut the door, went slowly to the fireplace, stooped down deliberately, stirred the fire.

"What is this little boy?"

"He is the cobbler's son."

"What is he doing here?"

"We have brought him along so he can hear some beautiful music. He has an excellent memory."

"That is a good trade, that of shoemaker."

I did not stir. I scarcely breathed. My legs were as heavy as if I had been hanged by my neck.

"The program!" demanded the woman.

Madame-la-Reine slowly straightened up.

In a voice which I did not recognize and which was like a prisoner he said, "My friend is going to sing:

> It is not lawful to put a man to death.
> Dissolve, O my heart, into torrents of weeping.

And:
> Help us, Christ, Almighty Son!

"These songs are parts of the Passion according to Saint John by Bach. The first and the last are chorals. My friend will sing the air only."

"And in the ancient manner," said the lady. "I do not pay you to give me a modern interpretation."

"Very well, Madame," said Madame-la-Reine.

He stepped forward to stand beside us and he drew his flute from the deep pocket of his coat skirt.

Just as the voice of the singer touched me with its iron wings, I perceived, in the shadow of the big armchair, a lower chair. It also was inhabited by a form which gradually became visible. It was a man who was either very old or very young. In the flickering light of the fire he grew young and then old without reaching a stationary age. Sometimes his hair was snow-white, then it seemed only blond, the blondness of baby hair. He had the head of a newborn baby, fat, white, soft, dead as those animal heads in the windows of the butcher shops, but in the very roundness of this head were etched the deep and dirty wrinkles of a sort of old age. The eye was not visible, or rather visible only in flashes in the swaying of this frightful head as big as a pumpkin. For the creature nodded its head ceaselessly; it seemed to be seeking with its nose some odor, some trace, some scent from which life might begin. At last it began to growl down in its throat like a little bull.

"Be quiet, Georges," said the lady.

At that very moment, or almost at that moment, a door opened in the dark end of the room. The odor of fried bacon and of burning grape-vine twigs entered. A woman asked, "Do you want the partridges rare?"

"The fat just golden brown," replied the lady without turning her head.

The door closed again.

Décidément was singing the great phrase:

"Lord, is it I who am to expiate the sins of men?"

It was no longer the imprisoned voice of Madame-la-Reine. It was the full voice, pure and free, which rose without effort from the very center of grief. There was no longer any politeness, any restraint, only freedom, and the grace and the force of the song were composed of that liberty in the lament. Even the flute was bantering and sorrowful. Behind the three of us who with our weakness of flesh and dress faced the great lady in silk with lips greased with partridge fat, all the inhabitants of our poor sheep court were wailing: the dark man who had lost his God, the naked girl, the Mexican woman who mourned her cactus, the little horse fed with old wood, the woman in the watery prison, my father, the beard of ferns that hung from the sink spout, the animal skins, the tanner who slept on a bed of salt. I heard in the heart of the music the wild voice of the anarchist as he went away toward Switzerland:

> The wretched will spring up about us like plants.

I was in the forefront of the battle.

When the song was ended, I no longer recognized Madame-la-Reine. He took two steps out of position.

"Is that not a harpsichord yonder, Madame?"

"Yes, it is," she said.

"Will you permit me to play, my friend accompanying with the violin, a little concerto of Christian Bach?"

He added after a short silence, "I think that it will give you pleasure."

"Do you know how to play the harpsichord?" said the lady.

"A little," he said.

"Where did you learn?"

Instead of answering he made a sign to Décidément, who obeyed in silence. Madame-la-Reine lowered the screw of the stool and sat down.

What followed, in its masterly skill, seemed to me so insolent that I took a step backward to hide in the shadow.

Then Madame-la-Reine gently shut the lid of the harpsichord.

"There," he said, "the Allegro, no more."

I do not know how we found our way out into the street.

In a little voice, measured, polite, exact, like the play of his fingers on the keys of the harpsichord, Madame-la-Reine sighed: "The main thing is to tell her to go to the devil."

"And to have her know we said it," added Décidément.

CHAPTER V

MY FATHER loved wounds and the sick. Old people would come to have him treat their eczema. He bathed it with a sedative water. The whole workroom smelled of camphor. He had finally rented a little piece of ground for twenty-five francs a year: ten meters of terrace on the ramparts of the town. It was fertilized with detritus and dirty water. A public washing pool ran over along its wall. There he cultivated rose bushes and hyssop. Sometimes he would take a rose between his two middle fingers, he would separate it from the stem without picking it, he would hold it on his hand, smell it, touch it, examine it.

"Job," he would say to me, "Job! He had great sores like this on his hands, on his feet, all over him. And he was as thin as a rail."

He loved epileptics. I mean, he gave them love. There was a big, redheaded one of whom I was afraid. He never shaved, and only cut his beard with scissors He was fat. He ate raw cloves of garlic all day long as one would eat candy. He was already a grown man and he had a tender affection for his mother, a little shriveled mouse with short legs and a long chicken neck deformed by a formidable Adams apple that ran up and down inside her neck like a very active chimney sweep at work in her throat.

He had a magnificent family name, Goliath. He went by his first name, Voltaire. Of his two brothers, one was called Tallien and the other Fabius. The father's skull was flat and the whole lower half of his face swollen by an enormous mouth bloodshot like a wound.

Voltaire was ashamed of his disease. Perhaps not precisely ashamed; he rather was haunted by it. He tried to put it out of his mind by doing the work of a well man. He was strong. He gave the impression of a man who was bearing a great sorrow and was trying to free himself of it by walking on a tightrope or juggling with torches. Then, he would fall down at any time or any place. The weight of this god that he bore in his head felled him near the hedge he had just begun to burn or by the stream where he was fishing for crayfish. That is how he was finally drowned.

When he was twenty he did not present himself in person at the board of examiners for military service. He did this on purpose. He was sent to the African Chasseurs. He was found several times lying under the feet of the horses in the stable.

"Don't tell," he would say.

He would treat to drinks. They didn't tell.

It was not out of patriotism. He detested the army. He was happy there because he was with all the husky fellows, the healthy ones, those whose brains were not shaking and enervated like caged panthers. One fine day, he fell off his horse during a review, at the moment when his squadron was galloping past the general.

"It must have been fatigue," my father told him, "all that bugle music, the heat—"

"No," said Voltaire, "it was the odor of my horse."

I have said that my father's workroom looked out onto a little court that belonged to a shepherd. From time to time sheep were parked down there. Finally the shepherd rented his court to a pork butcher who made a sty of it. He fattened his pigs with castoff milk and vegetables until the creatures could no longer budge, but lay in hollow places in the dung and the liquid which collected. It was only after the butchering that the straw was changed. The odor of the cleaning made Voltaire fall into one of his fits.

I said that I was afraid of this man. To be more exact, his first attack had made me want to vomit. The revulsion of my whole body had been so violent before the atrocious sight that I was left literally without bones or heart.

"Go get my pillow," said my father.

When I returned, he was wiping Voltaire's froth away with his own checked handkerchief. The man's head was bobbing about in my father's hands like a live creature. Sometimes it would escape and fall to the floor.

"Put the pillow under his head."

He looked at me. "It is nothing but a poor mechanical

thing," he said. "His brain has revolted. Go get Jules."

Jules was the butcher boy. I went down to the second floor in our own court. I called, "Jules!"

There was a little window in the wall opposite.

"Come over, my father wants you."

I waited there for him. The door of the corridor slammed. The soft tread of Jules, who had taken off his sabots, drew near.

"It's happened to him again," said my father.

Jules looked at the prostrate man. By dint of swinging the hammer to slay the oxen, Jules' shoulders and arms were swollen with fine fat red muscles. His bare chest was always visible beneath his buttonless shirt; a hairless chest, like woman's flesh. When my father changed his shirt, I could see his body cloaked with ram's wool from neck to waist, streams of black hair that sprang from his shoulders and ran to his hips. The nudity of Jules gave me a fearful thrill. Once I had seen him in the abattoir, naked to the waist. He was stationed before an ox. He had measured the distance by touching the ox's forehead with his outstretched left hand and he had swung the hammer.

"Help me," said my father.

Jules always took Voltaire by the feet. Even if upon coming in, he found himself near the sick man's head. He took two or three little soft steps and went and took him by the feet. My father put his hands under the poor man's armpits. He lifted him.

"Open the door, Jean."

Then I opened the bedroom door.

"He won't stir any more," said my father, "he is limp. He has entered his land."

Jules did not talk. He was puffing harder than when he carried great quarters of beef.

I said to myself: "Father is stronger than he."

They laid Voltaire on the bedside mat of goatskin. (I still have that bedside mat. This morning, before coming here to write these pages, I had set my bare feet once more on that gray hair that had been soft for the afflicted.) My father took off the blue comfort, drew down the sheet.

"Come on," he said bending down.

"With his shoes on?" asked Jules.

"Yes, leave them on him. We haven't time. He needs softness right now."

They laid the man in the bed. My father anchored the poor head by curving the coverlid around it.

"There!"

All was calm. We could hear our clock ticking.

"Haven't you anything to drink?" asked Jules.

"Yes, some Carmelite water."

Jules took the slender vial in his big fingers and he drank a long draught. His color came back.

"That's better," he said.

An hour later, when we returned from the workroom, my father said, "Sh!"

The door of our bedroom was softly creaking. A step crossed the landing, sought the stairs.

"It has passed, he is going."

Voltaire was leaving. Before going downstairs to supper, we went to make the bed.

"Don't say anything about it to your mother," my father said. "She would be frightened."

He smoothed the eiderdown with the palm of his hand; I could hear his skin rasping the old blue silk.

He added, "It would disgust her."

Sometimes he would say to me, "Go out on the landing and listen if they are singing."

It was dark. The depth of the court was ruddy because my mother's laundry had a window onto it. I listened:

"Yes, they are singing."

"Take the bottle of sedative water."

He was searching in the cupboard. He drew out some bath towels.

"Do you think these are any good?"

"Oh, yes!"

They were towels that were almost new. He sought some that were used.

"Come, don't make any noise."

We went downstairs. I carried the towels, he the bottle. Downstairs in the corridor he said, "Sh!"

We passed the door on tiptoes. My mother was softly singing the song of the "Golden Wheat."

My father had fixed the street door so it did not make any noise.

We went ten meters above where our house stood. We turned in under a dark cart arch.

"Follow the wall with your hand," he said.

The wall was all sticky and as if alive.

We went up a short flight, then down a corridor. At the end, you had only to push the door with your knee.

A heavy odor of urine stung my nose and throat.

A thick voice was chanting in the darkness: "The red horse! The red horse!"

The room smelled of the stable, old straw, liquid dung, saltpeter, and rotten wood.

"The red horse!"

There was no sound of movement, only the voice.

My father fumbled in his pocket for matches. Each time it was as if the red horse would emerge from the darkness at the crackling of the flame, in the tiny glow of phosphorus: the red horse, bare, scored with great roses, his bloody teeth revealed in laughter between his upturned lips.

Something scrambled in the straw; a rat flashed his two eyes.

The candle began to burn steadily. It revealed a form lying on a mattress.

"Come," said my father, and sometimes he would take my hand.

We entered the odor as through a woolen curtain; it was hot and it lay stifling against one's face. I swung my arms to ward it off.

"The rats have been here again."

My father was talking in his calm, contained voice. It was the same voice that said at table, "Pass me the bread, sonny."

"The rats have been here again."

Around the prostrate man my father had set traps, the kind that kill, and also cages.

There was one dead rat. There were two live ones in one cage and a third in another. The three live rats did not stir. Crouched in their prisons they watched with fixed eyes, and at the end of their little pointed noses, when they closed their mouths from time to time, their shiny little moustaches trembled.

"They have been eating again, the beasts!"

The man was covered with a coarse horse blanket, and under that, a sheet.

First it was necessary to lift the blanket.

The sheet was all spotted with great moist stains. My father drew the sheet off gently. Beneath each stain a wound clicked its open lips.

These wounds were alive. They were feeding on the paralyzed man, like the rats. The one on his stomach was enormous. It emitted a heavy carnivorous odor. He had two other wounds on his thighs.

"The towel."

I handed it to my father.

He poured out the sedative liquid.

"The red horse," chanted the man, "the red horse!"

He no longer felt even the sting of the alcohol.

"Look out," my father said to himself aloud. "That must hurt him."

He adjusted his spectacles.

"Well, it looks as if that was drying up a little."

The stomach wound was like a great bowl filled with

milk. The pus ran in tiny threads between the humps of flesh.

Before leaving, my father examined the man's shoulder.

"They have begun to eat here," he said.

He set the rat trap against the gnawed flesh. He took the other traps downstairs.

Below, in the darkness, I could hear my father put his hand into the wire cage. The rats began to squeal.

"One," said my father dully in his beard.

The rat was crushed against the wall.

"Two!"

"Three!"

Then he trampled them silently.

After every midday meal, my father would take a chair, carry it on his shoulder, and go off to his garden on the edge of town. He would sit between his two rose bushes. The pigeons from the convent would come and light on his shoulder.

CHAPTER VI

ONE EVENING as I was coming home from school (it was in November) it seemed to me all of a sudden that the boulevard smelled of violets. I stopped to sniff the air. Violets, but dreadful fleshy violets with quivering reddish flesh like the night that was descending over the bare branches of the elms. My throat hurt me. My books weighed in my arms. A buggy rushed swiftly by me. My eyes retained the movement of the horse's long white legs; I could not get rid of it, and as I rubbed my eyes to efface that image and restore the darkness, I realized that I was imitating with my mouth the clap, clap of the trot. I stopped it by shutting my lips tight. I told myself: "You'll have to stay up on your legs and keep on walking." My throat hurt me. A sound was following me like the darting buzz of a great fly. It would approach, filling my head with an iron-blue color in whose center the round eye of an oil street lamp glimmered like an almost extinguished firebrand; then it would recede with a brittle little sound, and my head was filled with a soft, syrupy yellow which slowly brought

silence and then again the November night on the boulevard and the odor of violets. I went toward the street of
the merchants that was lighted by the shops. It seemed to
me that this street was warm like an oven, that this evening I could, like the dogs, find in this warmth the different odors of all its inhabitants. I hugged my books tightly
in my arms. My throat was hurting me very badly. A
baker passed with a basket full of warm loaves on his head.
I realized that he turned his head to look at me and that
the whole basket had turned with his head, and that perhaps he had scattered all his loaves around him like a wet
wheel shedding drops of water. I could hear the loaves
enter the houses through the windowpanes, make a tour
of the rooms like russet birds, then alight on the cupboards
beside the clocks' round faces.

The fountain near the tobacco shop at the cross street
was making insolent sounds. I was thirsty and I began to
drink from the spout. The water ran down my neck. In
the basin of the fountain the reflection of the street lamp
caused a long golden hand to swim about, slender and
tapering. It wore a green ring. I thought that I must not
leave that ring there or the wife of the grave digger who
lived in this quarter would come with her pitcher; she
would spy the ring, she would take it and put it on her
own hand. I rolled up my shirt sleeve and fished in the
basin for the ring. It was easy for me to get it. It was a little
lettuce leaf. I opened one of my books with my wet hands
and carefully flattened the leaf between its pages. Then I
had to roll down my shirt sleeve, clasp my books tightly

under my arm, and go home. My throat hurt me and I had been unable to swallow the pain by drinking. The people were all walking bent over forward or to one side and several times I stopped because they were going to take just two or three more steps and then fall. No, they did not fall. They went on like that without knowing their danger. Near the church of Notre Dame the milkman had stopped. He had lifted his left knee, placed his jar on his knee and was pouring milk into a bowl that Mademoiselle Hortense was holding out to him. I heard her say "Good night," and then immediately there was no violet, nothing, only the sound of the milk was left in my head, and the sound of that woman's voice, the odor and the color of the milk, a white nothingness. And I was seized with a fierce desire for my mother, a need of my mama, of her arms, of her hand, and of her caress on my eyes. And this desire rose red and hot within me as if my heart had been heated at a forge.

When I opened our door, the smell of ironing was good. I just had time to notice the bowl in which the sprinkler was dipped.

"What is the matter with the child?" said my mother. "Look at him, he is sick."

As soon as one knows the interior passages of the air, one can depart at will from one's present and one's cares. One has only to choose the sounds, the colors, the odors which give the necessary transparence to the permeable air to dilate the pores of time and one enters time like an oil. For me, I need only a fire of dry twigs on the hearth, whitish weather with formless clouds, a little of that special wind that leaps in a ball like a partridge, a pipeful of coarse gray tobacco and I recapture the great shining rose window filled with distracted cries, which my mother's women-filled laundry became before my fevered eyes.

I must have collapsed against the table as I tried to clutch Louisa the First's apron.

I heard:

"My baby!"

"Vinegar!"

"Carry him!"

"Call his father!"

"My baby!"

Someone took me under my armpits and lifted me up. Antonine had opened the cupboard and was fumbling among the cruets. In the court someone was calling, "Père Jean! Père Jean!"

Then I heard him coming down the stairs. My mother rubbed my forehead moaning, "Good Lord! Good Lord!"

My father opened the door.

"The child!" said my mother. That was enough, and he bent over me while around his kind, distressed face, the whimpering faces of Antonine, the Louisas, and my mother whirled like a flock of birds in flight. My great worry was that green ring fished from the basin of the fountain. The pain in my throat I knew would go. My father was there with his bottle of sedative water. But the ring! The book would surely fall open. It was perhaps already in the sawdust and they would step on it and crush the lovely stone that was as big as a pea and break the tiny gold claws that held it. Then I knew that all was hopelessly lost.

"Take some hot stones up to his bed. I'll bring him up."

Father took me in his arms. Perhaps it was just as well, everything considered, for the green ring to go and flourish on the water-shriveled fingers of the grave digger's wife. I struggled no longer and the world burst like a sun.

Our bedroom looked out upon the sheep court. It is now dead and cold. A few months ago I went back to see it with some friends. There remains almost nothing of the grotesque paper with which it was decorated.

It was always evening. A bell was softly telling the hour. From the court came the monotonous drumming of the Mexican woman and her song that mounted like a bird call. Her voice rose in a falsetto and pierced the sky like a sharp white rasping knife cutting slices of the lowering sky. I had returned to the surface of life and was floating between two sheets: my face emerged only in the hollow of certain waves, but the water of mystery was no longer on my eyes save as a little transparent skin of liquid, and I could see the world, swollen and stiff, but still the world. However, it was always evening. My throat had been swabbed with a spoon wound with cotton. I clenched my teeth. They pinched my nose. I opened my mouth and they quickly probed down deep with the spoon handle and scraped my throat. Then I vomited pus, skin, and blood. Once I discharged from my nose two long candles of grayish membrane, throbbing and endowed with life like little wriggling fish. From that day, they let me alone, save to give me potent herb brews that descended inside me, hot, perfumed with the taste of earth and sun peculiar to irrigation waters in the summer meadows.

Little gilded corridors opened in the bedroom walls. All day long the bell told the hour. It never lost count but it was alone in giving any importance to the measure of time. The monsters on the wallpaper effaced their bellies with a slow movement, all together, and the little corridors opened. They went to the far reaches of the world. At precisely that moment everything out beyond must have been notified, and at once they all appeared. There was one creature who played a sort of soft flute, long as a snake. It would wind all about his body. And within it he played all his music. But the flute was silent. It only swelled up. Exactly like a snake that had eaten a bird. The music made a great bubble in the flute. Then the man would smile and pinch the hernia of music and the whole song would emerge with its largos and its trills, the whole song would emerge and shake its feathers and bathe in the dew, snap its beak, and fly away, a living thing. One minute I heard it strike its head against the ceiling, then it must have pierced it and it was gone. The Mexican woman was singing her "*Tapa mé, tapa méta pamé.*" There was also a creature of many breasts. They hung from every part, flapping about and spurting jets of milk or sometimes just drops until I finally hid my head beneath the covers. The creature loved the bedside mat. It would sit there and begin to graze on its long hair. From time to time this must have choked it and it would cough and open its great mouth and roll its tongue.

I also saw coming out of the wallpaper the somber heralds. I did not recognize them yet and from my sheet I would say softly, "Good day, Monsieur. Oh, what a lovely bell!"

But they would look at me with their cold staring round eyes, then they would strike their bells with their bony fists. I would listen politely to the strident sound as it disappeared down the long gilded corridors. Then these people jerked their heads like hens and their eyes blinked once as if to say, "It isn't possible, he does not understand! Let us wipe our eyes. It is not possible! Our bell! Our fist!"

Once more they became fixed and hard like mountains and they struck their bell again with their iron fists.

Before he went to fill his lamp, my father would come to see me. We were on the same floor, but before entering our bedroom it was necessary to pass through the "big room." He came over to my bed.

"Are you asleep?"

"No."

"Does it hurt?"

"No."

"How do you feel?"

"Better."

He would kiss me, and go away, leaving the bedside light turned low.

As soon as I was allowed to get up and go downstairs, I became the darling of the whole laundry full of women. They perfumed my handkerchief, gave me hard candies, tied the knot of my tie fifty times during the day, my tie that this time went round six times and rose to my ears and was cunningly stuffed with cotton inside. My mother had said, "And, when I go out, I'll kill anyone who does not look out for the child."

Those were fine winter days, warm and sweet, with a foretaste of lilacs; the twilight lasted all afternoon; it would swirl slowly over the hills like a great golden bird with blue feathers.

I said to Antonine, "I'm going out into the street a little."

"Yes, my sweetheart, go on out a little. They think you are made of sugar."

"But, undo this tie just a little."

And I had already begun to loosen it.

"No," said Antonine. "With the fright we've had, I am still sick at my stomach."

She tied my tie tightly and said, "I'm making you the secret knot."

And in fact she made me the secret knot that looked like a big snail and was hard as if made of dampened silk. It could never be undone.

Thus stiffly attired, I went up the street as far as the little rue des Paysans down which one went to the house of Décidément and Madame-la-Reine.

The house of the transients still smelled of martens and straw. The walls sweated a black grease, as sickening as sheep sweat. The door was open. I listened in the stairway. There was no sound of music. Décidément and Madame-la-Reine had gone out. Someone opened a door upstairs. I could hear a grave voice saying:

"Don't stay too long. Just look and see if there are

people in the café. And above all, don't drink anything, please, don't take anything to drink. Come back quickly, my darling. We aren't in such need as that. I am afraid by myself."

"You are afraid?" asked the little voice of the girl who bathed naked in front of the window.

"Yes, I am afraid when you are not here," replied the man.

They continued to talk in low tones, then there was a moment's silence. I could not hear them speak or move.

At last she started down. The slow, grave voice came down behind her.

"Don't be long, darling."

She stopped on the landing.

"Just the time it takes," she said, "if someone wants it. If not, I'll come right back."

He shut the door up there and this time she came on down, hopping from one foot to the other with her wooden-heeled boots.

She found me on the doorsill.

"What are you doing here?" she said.

I did not answer. I looked at her. She was powdered white and her lips were like raw flesh. She smelled of musk.

She sat down on the doorstep. Her face was on the level with mine.

"Whistle your tune for me," she said.

It was evident that she wanted it badly. She moistened her lips with the tip of her tongue and her eyes blinked gently like a bird about to take flight.

"Whistle."

But I could not whistle and I told her that I had been sick.

"So that is why we haven't seen anything of you," she said. "And who tied your tie? That must hurt you, it is too tight."

She put her hand on the secret knot and before I could warn her that it was a secret knot, it was undone. She had knowing hands.

"Wait."

And she softly rolled the silk about my neck. She was careful to give it fine folds, I felt that.

"Wait."

She unrolled one whole turn to do it better, and at last she fastened the two little ends in a simple solid knot that spread with a pinch of her fingers into two butterfly wings.

"There!"

Then she gave me a kiss. This made several times that I had met her since the funeral of the acrobat's little girl. At first she had said to me, "Hello, little boy."

Then she had touched my cheek with the tip of her finger, then she had kissed me.

She had a kiss that was sweet, warm, good.

When I had heard her coming down the stairs just now, I had hoped for that.

She stood up. She went off.

She stopped in front of the little café, Au Tonneau, and looked in through the glass. I could hear them calling to her inside. She put her hand on the doorknob, gave me a tired, gentle little smile, and went in.

I returned to the laundry. My mother had not yet come back.

"You have touched your tie, monster," said Antonine.

And as she was retying it, she added, "He's a demon, this child. He smells of musk. He has been letting the hussy kiss him again."

Saturday was the day of the animal fair and the creatures were sold inside the town. On the eastern boulevard they herded the pigs, and on the western boulevard where the morning coolness remained, where the ramparts lulled a morning shade, pricked with sharp dew, they made the horses run. This place sparkled with kicks and neighs, and all the echoes of the walls trembled as in a thunderstorm. There was not a doorstep that did not ring with the sound of whips and gallopings. The horse dealers drank standing, leaning against the elms, or sitting on the huge roots that protruded from the ground. The sheep slept in the squares in the interior of the town, in the lovely cool and calm. The winter sun never came there to these tiny fountain squares. There was always a little café for the shepherd in one corner. The odor of sheep flowed down the sloping streets. It descended gently like mortar; it stopped at the joiner's; it butted its nose against the scent of dead pines; it ran a little farther down to the baker's, to greet the taste of fagots and bran that throbbed with the reflection of the flames in front of the oven's open jaws; it touched the bared teeth of the raw salt piles on the doorsills of the tanneries. It went on all alone, then it met the odor of the pigs, then it met the odor of manes and tails plaited with red straw, the odor of sweating mares and the terrible scent that the stallions gave off in heavy sprays as they neighed to the imprisoned females. Then all that together billowed in great waves and rose from the street gratings to the heavens. All the winter birds were appalled by it and they fled to the hills crying sadly, as though the end of the world was near.

The shepherd, Massot, came to the house to eat his lunch, a great noonday lunch of bread and meat well washed with wine. He chewed long and slowly in order to taste everything; the bread by itself, the meat by itself, the meat and bread mingled, and he always drank before finishing his mouthful to add to the taste.

On these days, the inns cooked great caldrons of beef stew, and when it was one of those dry winter days with open sky, hard and round beneath the sun like granite stones in the river bed, this stew was served outdoors on long trestle tables. All the animal dealers lined up by clans or by villages and they began to mop up the gravy with hunks of bread. They stood before the bench, they took the dipper and poured dippersful of stew into deep dishes. For they were given soup plates, broad and deep, like crows' nests. And so, from the very beginning of the afternoon, when they all settled down, in the sun, to digesting and belching in their moustaches, an odor more terrible than that of the penned-in creatures rose to terrify the fleeing birds, and then the sky became still as death.

This particular day, Père Massot did not wear his peasant blouse.

"I dressed myself like a bourgeois," he had said when he came, "and besides I've come in the cart."

He had not come to market. He had not brought his big stick embellished with knife carvings, copper nails, and leather thongs, and this gave his hands a blank look; they looked stupid without employment. He had spent the morning with my father.

At noon, I understood that the affair concerned me.

Père Massot looked me over.

"He looks pretty seedy," he said.

My mother explained the situation to me.

"You need the country. It will bring your health back. Here you hardly eat a thing, and besides it is too hot or too cold. Madame Massot will take good care of you. If you get homesick, they will bring you back. Père Massot will bring you with him every Saturday."

What my father said to me was rather different and I did not understand much except that he was very moved and glowing inside, as it were, with a sort of quivering, uneasy joy like a fire that asks only a breath of wind to cause it to burst into flame.

He talked to me of sheep and the country, of grass and trees.

"Oaks," he said.

I remember that as he said that he expanded his chest and his beard began to flutter softly.

"You are never to go to the stream. There is a very deep hole in it and children have been drowned in it. You'll see, the threshing floors are like the prow of a ship. You'll see, the hill is all covered with huge juniper bushes that look like monks. You'll have to look at it all and get your own picture of it for yourself. As I have done. As everyone ought to do. You will have to learn to live with little comrades, too. That is the school for later on in life. Eat Madame Massot's soup nicely. It is coarse soup, but it is just because it is coarse that it will teach you to see things as a whole. And get some muscle. Big shoulders are useful in life, even if it is only to pull a thorn out of a hand."

And so on until at last the fire was all alight in him and I had ripened into a human being in its glow like a great round loaf.

He talked to me a little longer, then he looked at the shepherd, Massot, and said to him, "I give him into your keeping."

The shepherd sat a moment calculating, then he laid his hand on my arm.

"I'll take him for you," he said.

They each realized their responsibilities, and they accepted them.

The shepherd Massot lived at Corbières. It took two hours to reach it in the cart, the horse trotting all the way. We passed Sainte-Tulle, we went around two hills, and suddenly we were confronted by a high wall of earth and rocks. The threshing floors. They dominated the whole valley like a great nest. Behind them, the village lay along the side of the hill. Thus it was sheltered from the wind and had reserved for the wind a vast flat piece of ground where its dull stamping could be heard before it set off again. Thanks to this wind, Corbières had the cleanest grain in the whole valley, and when they winnowed on the threshing floor, the people way on the other side of the valley, in the little village of Vinon, had to shut their windows, for they were assailed by great swarms of chaff. The swallows called to each other from town to town; the goldfinches left the woods; the cardelines devastated the bushes as they flew through them like mad creatures, and all these birds fluttered and shrilled in the flying grain dust. Sometimes the goshawks and shrikes slid gently from a fold in the clouds and darted down to strike the sparrows. The hoopoes came up from the swamps and the sky battle burst with such fury that it drowned the sounds of the winnowing machines. Dead sparrows were picked up in the roads and at night the crows did not go to sleep in the church steeple. They gathered in the hollow of the high bell and spent the whole night in a wild dance, emerging intoxicated from the holes, chasing the owls clear down to the willows by the stream, scratching on the stones of the church with such fury that the scraping of their claws was audible.

That is what winnowing on the Corbières threshing floors was like.

We reached there one calm evening. The red winter was still on the hills. The baker was cleaning his oven and we had to cry "Whoa!" to the horse and stop, for every time the baker drew out his long shovel, he had to cross the street. At last he let us pass. He came to the threshold. He had the chest of a bull, a moustache that turned up into his nose, and two eyes like loosely attached globes.

"So you've brought the little one," he said.

There I was, wrapped in my cloak and filled with ecstasy. On the square they were burning dead gorse and the village rose, living, from the smoke. Houses in which lamps were lighted winked their eyes. The church tower lifted its arm; it had lace at the cuff and its slim hand was trying to show me the vast sky overhead. Yes, above was only the advancing night, the early winter night still bloody with cold, but it was more alive than the night that I used to see from the window of my father's workroom. This one had gently laid its green belly over the fixed motion of the hills like a great bird (its irritated claws still scratched the setting sun), and it spread its wings over the whole sky, covering it all, soothing it with the slow fanning of its plumes. Its wings covered the world to the farthest mountains and, for the first time, like a little mountaineer, watching the motionless tide of the highlands fall asleep before my eyes, I began to tremble as I imagined the nightfall on the sea.

The fastening had indeed been broken; the seal had burst and the doors opened wide. Doors no longer existed, the threshold was passed, I was in the vast land of the winds.

Madame Massot received me with clasped hands. It was only after having sighed deeply, admired profoundly, carefully weighed with her eye, and smacked her lips in advance over all the kisses she wished to give me, that she decided to stoop over me. She rubbed my nose, my cheeks, and my mouth, and called me "My partridge!"

She was an agreeable country lady, very ugly; with so much goodness in her blind eye, so much goodness in her good eye, so much goodness in her moustache, in her snuff-taking nose, in her sagging cheeks, in her black-lipped mouth, that she was frightfully ugly. It was an ugliness made of all that sacrifice, of all that martyrdom which constitutes real goodness. In the photograph that I saw in the bedroom where she was holding in her hand the forefinger of the shepherd Massot, all rigged out for the wedding, she was beautiful and fresh and seemingly inflated with an artless loveliness. That creature had to be gradually broken, burned, twisted, kneaded; the eye blinded, the body made ungainly, be cooked in the oven of goodness like a brick or a pot; it had to forget everything but that little red fruit that was the heart. She had fully succeeded.

There were fritters, bilberry jam, warm goat's milk with hair in it, a piece of toast rubbed with garlic, a moment's pause in front of the crackling hearth, then a bed, all warmed by a hot stone, that was hard, hot, and scented with lavender like the bed of a summer stream.

Sleep came in three easy leaps while I was murmuring, "Why did they put her eye out, I wonder."

There was a meadow, and in this meadow, a fig tree. I used to climb up to where the branches made a cradle. I would call softly, "Anne!"

She was almost always sitting among the reeds. I would call once, twice at the most: her face would emerge from the earth. She was thin, pale, dark, with huge black eyes, and her lips that I was constantly touching with the tip of my finger burned like live coals. She would come and sit beside me.

"In the snake," she would say.

But I was the one who had taught her that. I was the one who had said, "The branches of the fig tree are like a big angry snake, but it coils to make a basket of itself for little children."

And then I had taught her to play "lost boat." It was enough to have a stream and a bit of wood. We had the stream; it was the tiny meadow brook. There it was all alone with its poor scaleless water. It would twist among the stones and you had to blink hard to discover, in the place of the streamlet, a great river from beyond the seas.

Anne knew how to blink exactly as I did and she saw the river.

We took a piece of wood that floated easily, a bit of cork bark or a sliver of a stick.

"There are five on it," I said.

"Five?" asked Anne, raising to me her big eyes of milk and coal.

"Yes, five: a big fellow with a beard, he's the chief. A little one with boots, he's the one who carries the revolver. A skinny one who carries the guitar slung over his shoulder, the faithful Mastalou, and the captive maid."

"Who is the captive maid?"

"A little girl."

"What's she like?"

"Alive."

I meant that she was alive and bound with leafy vines and that the men were carrying her away.

And we gave the wood to the waters of the stream, and the boat went off down the river with the guitar, the revolver, the beard, the Negro's laugh, and the little girl's moans, because the vines bound her too tightly.

We followed the adventure step by step.

Sometimes the company slipped through the pouring oil of a rapid; at other times the boat plunged down a waterfall, or it got caught in some quicksand of a muddy shore and would stay there shivering, powerless and trapped.

It was forbidden to touch it. We could only watch and let fate do her work.

"Just once," said Anne.

"No."

"They'll die."

"That's too bad."

"Only the tip of my finger."

"No."

And I would pull Anne swiftly toward the fig tree. We would stay there, silent, looking into the short winter grass, absorbed by the winding valley of a great mysterious river.

"Who knows where they are now?" said Anne.

"That's their lookout."

Fate has her work all laid out. She has arisen before us. She says: I'll do this, this, and this. And she does it.

Spring came upon us with two or three blasts of icy wind. The tip of my nose froze and thawed, froze and thawed, and I did as the other little country boys do: I ran my warm tongue over my upper lip. My hands were blue with cold. Then the weather began to purr and to play with the earth with its claws half-sheathed, like a cat playing with a ball of wool. Sometimes you could feel the claw, at others, the warm softness of fine deep fur, perfumed with animal sweat. Finally it scratched beneath the trees and the flowers came out; it raked the meadows and the little frogs began to peep; it split the hills, the nightingales flew away and it was spring.

One evening, about five o'clock, while there was still a little daylight, they brought home the wheelwright's son. Four men carried him. They had laid him on a ladder. The four men walked silently with their free arms extended, less because of the weight than to push aside the night.

"Mille!" they cried.

As they laid the body on the ground, night fell. The wheelwright came out of the forge. He could not see by dint of his eyes being filled all day long with fire, and he asked softly, "What? What's the matter?"

The son had broken his back. He had fallen asleep on the cart. It was only by chance that he was found on the deserted road near Mirabeau.

He remained alive that night, and the next day. His mother watched over him in silence. Madame Massot stayed there in the room to await the moment, and I, from the shadow where I was, saw the son lying still under his sheet, and through the door, in his father's room, on his father's bed, the Sunday clothes ready and waiting, too.

The father had gone down to the shop. He stayed there all day making horseshoes.

They said to him, "Stop it, nobody needs them."

"*I* need them," he replied. And he continued to forge—for himself.

Toward evening the son asked, "What time is it?"

"Six o'clock," said Madame Massot.

"Help yourselves," said the boy.

The two women looked at each other.

"What does he mean? What do you mean, Charles?"

He was dead as they looked at each other.

There were two days' respite. Three. It was a Thursday evening when they buried the boy, and it was the following Sunday, after the ball, that young Costelet shot himself with a gun in the lower jaw.

Thursday the wind jostled the procession on the way to the cemetery; it took stones from the ground and threw them on the box. The curé turned around two or three times to see who did it. Friday, a wind like water, a wind that touched everything; no time to breathe. I believe that Mélanie was the only one all day long who crossed the village street. Only Mélanie; she opened the door, she crossed over to Hortense's house. To talk. On Saturday, then, the wind was at its height; the body of the wind. Until then, we had had only the ends of its hair, the tips of its fingers, the arms of the driving wind. Now it came on the village with the force of its shoulders, and up in the hills you could see that its belly had touched the earth and was plowing up the fields. On that day no one ventured out, and all day there was that long "whooo" in one's ears. Massot was beside the hearth, his head in his hands. From time to time he would press his little finger in the tunnel of his ear and shake it. And on Sunday, after a whole night when everything rang—walls, belfry, bells, the church, the tin roof of the washing pool, trees, the whistling stones of the ramparts—Sunday dawned, very simply, with its sun, its great sky robed like the Holy Virgin, and a peace and a silence in which the steps of the ants could be heard.

After that, the ball.

Costelet's sweetheart, everyone knew, was Germaine. She danced five dances with him. She danced one dance with Vernet of Plombières. Costelet turned his attention to Marguérite du Bachas. They could be heard laughing. Germaine tried to look into the shadow. She could not see what they were doing. They weren't doing anything. We had seen them, Raphael and I. During the ball we played hide-and-seek and I was hiding behind the bench. No. Costelet was sitting looking over at his Germaine yonder. From time to time he would say a word without moving, and Marguérite would laugh because one must laugh when one is with a boy in the dark. And she was laughing just to laugh, little nervous giggles deep down in her throat.

Germaine came up to them.

"You are coming?"

"No, go with your Vernet."

She danced once more, then she sat in a corner all alone.

Costelet crossed the dance floor without glancing at her. He went out and around back of the church to his house. He took the gun, went up on the threshing floors to the straw stack, where he and Germaine used to go in the evening, where the hollow they had made was still in the straw, and he shot himself through the head.

After the ball, Germaine found him.

This time there was little peace. The gendarmes came. They went and examined the straw stack.

"What is that?"

The fat gendarme had found a little ribbon.

"Nothing."

"And yet!" said the gendarme.

And he held the ribbon bow in the palm of his huge hand.

Yes, he was right, everything was there.

Julie Costelet began to wail as soon as the body was in the box. They had nailed it shut early because the weather was warm.

"I didn't say anything," said the carpenter to Madame Massot, "and nobody must say anything about it, but his head had already begun to smell, and there was a worm in his eye."

Julie Costelet began to wail. That lasted like the north wind, day and night, without respite. The wail reached me in my bed. It made the globe of the clock tremble. I got up softly. I put a folded piece of paper under the globe to keep it from rattling. I went back to bed. The noise was still there beside the cry. It took me a long time to discover that it was the glass of a photograph that was gently shivering between the picture and the frame. I laid the photograph flat on the marble and the cry remained alone. It was like a long panting that never stopped. I buried myself under my covers. There was no connection, but there, in my bed, besieged by that long, heavy moaning, I could see clearly in the darkness before me the face of the girl with the musk, the girl who had kissed me in the street. I saw especially her look, something so simple and frank, and deeply wounded. I remembered also all the monsters of my fever during my illness. For a while I saw the great colored birds coming through the night with their big eyes shining like wet boxwood, the heavy, many-breasted pachyderms of a violet color, bristling with nails and horns. During that time I could no longer hear Madame Costelet's wailing, and then suddenly, it pierced these visions like a stone in the reflection on still water, and it tore and broke and effaced everything that it might be all alone, a wailing as naked, in its simplicity, as a knife. It was alone, then deep within it shone the face of the girl with the musk. That may have had some connection.

They said to Madame Costelet, "Shut up! What good does that do you?"

She was silent a moment. "None," she said, "none."

And on Wednesday morning, a week after the death of Charles, the wheelright's son, Justin, who was setting out at the crack of dawn with his cart, found the fat baker hanging from the first linden on the highroad.

He came back to tell the village and I heard his voice. I went to the window. He was down below in the white light of dawn, and he was calling:

"Clodomir, Monsieur Tastu, Fine, Olivier, Massot!"

Every time he called Massot, he turned toward our house a face in which all was blotted out save a mouth open wide in his beard.

I went and pulled at Madame Massot's hand. It was hanging down outside the cover.

"I hear," said the shepherd.

Then Madame Massot woke up.

"What?" she said.

"This is probably going to keep up," said the shepherd.

"Costes has hanged himself," shouted Justin.

"Costes," said Massot. "I knew it. He was marked."

The curé preached a special sermon. Monsieur Tastu took his cane and went through the village. He rapped on the doors with the knob of his cane. The doors opened.

"Good day, Monsieur Tastu."

"Good day, Fine, or Clorinde, or Chabassut, good day. Well, how's everything?"

They would look out at the springtime without replying.

"Well," said Monsieur Tastu, "it's a disease, it can be cured. We'll have a festival Sunday."

"No one has the heart for it."

"We must," said Monsieur Tastu, "we can make the effort. The medicine comes later. It is inside, and this will help. Get out of yourselves."

"As you like."

During the week, Blanche Lamballe hanged herself to an olive tree with her belt. She hadn't any reason. They found her in the morning. The night wind had played with her and had stolen her skirt. She was clad only in her blouse and her linen slip which did not even cover her thighs.

We were going to play in Pierrisnard's little pasture; Raphael, Louis, Anne, Mariette, Pierre, Turc, and I. It was an abandoned garden beside the village. There was nothing in it but nettles and brambles, and if we played at digging in the sand of the bank, we had to scratch carefully because the salamanders were sleeping their winter sleep in this sand.

"Do you want us to hang you?" said Raphael.

"Yes."

He put his leather belt around Mariette's neck. They hoisted the little girl up to the branch. They hanged her. She fell into the nettles, coughed, and vomited. She looked at us with big troubled eyes.

"I saw the blue," she said.

"What's it like?"

"You shut your eyes and your whole head fills with blue."

Anne never wanted to go home with us, but would stay all by herself in the path and then she would go off toward the hollow where the stream was.

One evening we had to run after her and call, "Anne! Anne!"

We found her lying prone and trembling in the reeds.

On Friday morning the curé went from house to house.

"Put out your fires," he said.

They began to extinguish their hearth fires and they threw the matches into the basin of the fountain.

The curé opened the great double door of the church. To open the left side required the strength of three men.

He said Mass all alone inside.

While he was doing this, the people laid little bundles of lavender and dried thyme on their hearths.

About ten o'clock, the curé came out of the church, bearing a lighted taper. With his wax taper he rekindled all the fires.

"We have new fire," said Madame Massot, "that's what we need."

And she sprinkled the flames with coarse salt which began to sputter and explode like little thunderbolts.

In the afternoon, the curé saddled his horse and went to the town to get matches for everyone.

And on Sunday there was a festival. The streets were decorated with box and flowering almond branches. The town crier made his rounds quietly and early. Wardrobes were opened. One had to wear one's Sunday best. At the hour for Mass, the curé came out once more into the sunlight, but he himself was like a sun: his gold cape was embroidered on the front with the lamb holding its cross between its little feet. The cold ashes of the old fires had been preserved. The curé walked at the head of the others to the ramparts of the threshing floors. The wind on that day was strong but without caprice and it had turned its course and hollowed its bed in the direction of the sea. The people advanced to the ramparts and emptied the sacks of ashes into the wind.

Costelet's Germaine cried out, "My sun! My sun!"

And she struck her head against the stones. They carried her away. She was whinnying like a mare.

They danced in front of the church. The wheelwright

and his wife sat on chairs and watched the dancing. Germaine came with her face ravaged from tears and she danced. She danced with a different man each time. She did not talk. She did not try to recover her balance by reversing from time to time as girls do; no, she whirled like a top until she was dizzy. And each time the music stopped, her partner had to support her and push her to the bench. As soon as the music started up again, as soon as the trombone player began to beat time, Germaine stood up and advanced toward a man, arms outstretched, so that he had only to seize her by the waist and bear her off.

It ended about midnight. They helped the café proprietor take in his benches and trestles. Soon no one remained under the lamp but Monsieur Tastu, the curé, and Massot. Down by the threshing floors there was singing: a chorus of boys and girls.

"That's better," said Massot; "we must keep it up."

Once I saw a snake at very close range. I have never been afraid of snakes. I love them as I love weasels, martens, partridges, hares, little rabbits, everything that does not have the association of death or the hypocrisy of love. Snakes are wonderful, peaceful, and sensual creatures, born in the very heart of the earth, in the place where the essence of granite, basalt, and porphyry must lie; they are indeed of an extraordinary beauty and grace.

This snake had appeared almost under my foot. It had darted, like a fish, and it was fleeing. There was nothing on the hill but crushed rocks; no grass, no tufts of thyme; it could not hide. It was not going fast. The sinuous move-

Blue Boy

ments of its body did not make a track in the dirt and it dissipated its strength in its contortions without making much headway. It was as thick as my arm. It heard me walking deliberately behind it, and then it reared on its sickle-curved tail. Gently it swayed its head from side to side. It had great green muscles that rippled the length of its body. It hissed in its throat like a kitten, and darted out its tongue. It looked at me. Its eyes were round, full, and cold like a bird's. I could see its anger, its fear, its curiosity rising beneath its skin, and perhaps also a little of that tenderness which, I learned later, all snakes have for men. I was a very little man. I saw chiefly its fear and its anger. It was like grass smoke rising up inside it; its anger was green and slightly gleaming like foam; as it mounted it made its scales click. Its fear was a blue ripple that ran within the anger. There were little flashes of red the whole length of its body. They would light up and then go out like tiny coals. They were under the scales. There was a brilliant yellow like the sun and a dull yellow of light clay, and a still, metallic yellow, and all these colors fused the length of it and all over it.

It stopped hissing. It was looking at the world with something cold and dead. Its eyes were only a mechanism. All its sensitivity was in its skin and its flesh.

I often used to imagine things as lovely as the skin of a serpent. The coldness of its eyes, the dead look in its eyes, I have never seen save in the eyes of Costelet when he went to get his gun, and in the face of the girl perfumed with musk.

I had never seen it anywhere but there.

But the snake, like a flow of water turned off, lowered its body, as if reassured, and went slowly off among the stones.

And now, on my way back to the village, as I entered the streets I found these dead eyes in nearly everyone.

Anne had seen Costelet's wound. She had lifted the cloth while the dead man was still lying in the straw and scarcely cold. Then softly she had retreated a step, and gone away with a finger on her lips as if to impose silence.

She said to me, "The angel that was in his head spread its wings to fly away and broke his head."

I thought about that angel in the vegetable shed. I often used to go there to hide, all alone, away from everyone. I would hear Madame Massot calling, "Jean! Jean! Where can he be?"

She talked to herself.

"It's time for *goûter*. Bilberry jam!"

She would close the jar and put it back in the cupboard. And I would not answer. I could hear the bilberry jam escaping from me. I wanted it very much. I would not answer. I would stay hidden, huddled in a ball between two sacks of potatoes.

The angel!

I was thirteen years old. I felt that I had an angel, too, like everybody else; like the snake. For every time that I thought about the angel, I would remember the enflamed surge of anger and fear through the snake's body. I felt that this angel was at that moment seated in my head between my ears; that it was there, alive, and that all my joys came from these two facts: that it was *there* and *alive*. I felt that it was like the snake's, made of the ability to be afraid, of the capacity for anger, curiosity, joy, of the power of tears, of the fact of existing in the world, penetrated by the breath of the world, as a drop of water suspended in a ray of sunlight is ablaze because of its translucency.

The angel!

It is the child of our flesh. It is molded by the hands of God: yes, and by our own. All those keen little hands of our eyes and ears, all those sensitive little hands by which our blood touches the world, as a child touches an orange; those little burning hands of our lips, the black hand of our spleen, the purple hand of our liver, the broad hand of our lungs, the musician hand of our heart, the laborer in mortar that toils in our belly, and the maker of wings that flaps gently like a fish between our legs, or throbs like a warm little frog: these are our hands.

And the angel is there, quietly seated at the summit of our neck, between our two ears.

"It spread its wings to fly away and broke his head." Sometimes the head is too hard.

One Saturday, Massot hitched up the two-wheeled cart.

"Let's go and see your papa."

My father was bent over an old shoe. He held it tightly against him and was cutting the edge of the sole with his knife.

He was humming in his beard.

"Satisfied?" asked Massot.

"No!" said my father.

He examined me with pleasure. *His* eyes were not dead, the life in them was only tired.

"You must not waste your time," he said, "and you have not wasted it. I am pleased with your shoulders. Let's see your arms. They'll do. Lift those anvils there in the corner."

He watched me lift and move the two masses of iron.

"That's fine," he said, "now look at me. Good. That's all right. You have not wasted your time there either. Only you must grow a little more in that direction. Massot, you must keep the boy for me all this spring, all summer, but bring him back to me every Saturday and let him stay here all day. He will go back to school in October. Sonny, open the trunk yonder. There's a package of books in it. They were given to me for you. The man said that you were to begin to read the first one. Next Saturday he will be here. You are to tell him what you have not understood, he will explain it to you. So. And now, go drink your *café au lait*."

As soon as I was out on the stairs I untied the string and opened the package. There was the *Odyssey*, Hesiod, a little Vergil in two volumes, and a Bible bound in black.

Downstairs, the laundresses had arrived. My bowl of *café au lait* was served on the ironing table.

"Your sweetheart is dead," Antonine told me.

The mouthful of *café au lait* became hard as a stone in my mouth.

"She used to kiss you, she gave you her odor."

I went back up to my father's room. My heavy country shoes scraped on the sandstone steps. I recalled the light

little step of the girl with the musk as she descended her
stairs, the slipping of her hand along the wooden banister,
and the sound of the big silver ring that struck against the
banister when she took hold of it below the post, the frou-
frou of her skirt, and the little hop of her two feet on the
flagstone at the bottom.

"What are you doing here?"

Powdered white, red of lips, bare armed, her blouse open
to the shadow.

The man upstairs had said before letting her go down,
"Don't stay long. I am afraid when you are not here."

I opened the door. My father was working in silence.
Massot was reading a letter. I went and looked out of the
window. Over there where she used to bathe every morning it was all shut up. There were no towels drying on
the line.

Massot folded the letter.

"Yes," he said, "you could send that one too. I think it is
very good, Père Jean." And he handed him the letter.

"I know that it is good," said my father. He put the
letter into his drawer.

Here is the letter. I have it here before me, with many
others. I copy it.

Monsieur,

I thank you for all you have done for Marie-Louise. She
told me not to forget. She told me again before she died. You
have given all, and more, that a living soul can give another
living soul. You brought her tranquility and peace. I must
thank you for the care with which you had her honorably
buried. I cannot repay you the forty francs which you lent

me. I am giving you these books for your son. They are not worth forty francs and I would not dare to offer them to anyone but you. As to the plan about which you talked to me: to give lessons to your son every Saturday, I cannot agree to it before telling you about myself. You do not know me. I am honest, and before accepting, I must tell you who I am. I should have come to see you and talked about all this. You will excuse me if I prefer to write it. I am thus separated from that goodness that emanates from you and for which I am so hungry that it might perhaps force me to lie. I know, on the other hand, that I owe you forty francs and I might be tempted to acquit myself by giving lessons to your son. It would not be honest to do it before giving you every bit of information about myself. Excuse me for writing this to you.

I cannot tell you my story, Monsieur. I am going to tell you that of a friend. We were at the Seminary together and we were the same age. He was at first the servant of a mountain hamlet, then he had the curacy of a village in the marshes. I often went to see him. In the springtime, the water came up into the streets, then it would recede and the white down of the reeds would fly in the air like dust. In the winter, he warmed himself with moldy willow logs. The odor of that makes you old.

He had an uncle in Lyons, rich and ill, who died, making him his heir. A little inheritance: six thousand francs; the rest went to religious orders. Toward the end of his life, the uncle had been tended by a young nurse. My friend went to Lyons. He had to go. In the first place, to thank the memory of this uncle who owed him nothing and left him six thousand francs, and then to get the money. My friend longed for a horse. He could thus cross the ford whenever he wanted to and go riding in the hills all afternoon. The uncle was already buried and he found the young nurse, sick, consumptive, and in bed. The house was to go to the Dominicans. The young girl had to get out as quickly as possible. They had allowed her several days longer through the charity of the Prior. She had reached that stage where not even a dog would have the courage to force her to get up and walk. My friend took his money, paid for a carriage and the journey, and took the young girl home with him. He was twenty-five years old. He made a room for her next to the kitchen. It got the heat from the kitchen stove. He left the door open and he could talk with her as he worked at the table under the lamp or as he prepared the meals. It was necessary to get medicine. But my friend had not bought himself the horse, and with six thousand francs one can buy medicine. He tried a little of everything. The young girl was very gentle. Gentle, and full of tenderness and gratitude. She softly called him "Monsieur le Curé." There was nothing secret. The women of the village came to see the sick girl. In all the houses they said, "I have been to see the curé's wife." I assure you that they said this without malice, with no evil thought, as you would say it yourself, Monsieur.

This lasted for two years. Then she died. Toward the end, he would often spend the afternoon at her side. He would sit with his back against the light. He would take the young girl's hand in his and they would remain thus, the two of them. They did not talk. They did not stir. Just the touch of the fingers, and then with his hand in hers. After that, Monsieur, they did not stir. She died without him, all alone, her blood spilled on the sheets. When he returned, she had been cold for a long time. He buried her in the village. He said the Mass for the dead. The cemetery was full of water.

When he came back from the cemetery, my friend opened his trunk. Inside were a hunting coat and trousers. He took off his cassock, he dressed himself as a layman. He locked the church and he went away.

That happened to my friend fifteen years ago. Since then, he has been in many places.

You asked me to find out why they would not receive Marie-Louise in the town hospital. You will excuse me for not telling you why before this. You will excuse me especially for having thought that that might prevent you from doing what you have done for her. I cannot forgive myself for having thought this now that I know what you are. When I went to see the mayor, he told me that the hospital was run by the good Sisters, that Marie-Louise was tattooed all over, and that it was not a spectacle for the good Sisters. He told me that Marie-Louise had a serpent tattooed on one leg, that it wound around her thigh and that it plunged its head higher up, in the obvious place. Excuse me, that is what he told me, and it was true.

Thank you again, Monsieur. I shall never forget what you did for her, for the sound of your voice when you talked to her, and that you kissed her twice, once when she was alive, and once when she was dead.

CHAPTER VII

With the end of spring, we had a new guest. He arrived at Massot's house one evening. He gently greeted us at the threshold.

"Is this Monsieur Massot's house?"

"Yes."

"Monsieur Jean sent me."

"Come in."

He entered. He moved very quietly. Over the sound of his living rose the loud buzzing of the gadflies and wasps in the flowering honeysuckle.

It was the dark man.

Outside, the great heat had already eaten the whole surface of the earth to the depth of a hand's breadth and the wind was clad in a thick, heavy, woolly dust that swept through the trees with the roar of fire.

The man looked as if he had just come through a long rain. His hat hung about his head as if it were soaked, and when he removed it, his thin, limp hair drooped over his forehead. He was afraid of bothering people.

"I am in your way," he would say, starting up from his chair.

"Stay where you are," said Madame Massot.

And then Massot, who was paring an ax handle with his knife, stopped and looked up.

"You aren't in anybody's way," he said. "That's just a habit you have of saying that, and it gives a bad impression. There is room for everybody here. If there isn't room, I say, 'Sit outside.' I told you to come in. That was to make you welcome inside. You will see. Take off your coat, roll up your shirt sleeves and come with me. I've been wanting to move the bread trough, and since you are here. . . ."

They placed themselves one at each end of the trough.

"Take care," said Massot, "it is heavy. I have been waiting for a man to come along. Have you got it?"

He took hold of it. He put all his strength into it. His arms trembled like ropes.

"A little more," said Massot.

Then:

"A little to the right."

Then:

"Close to the wall. Nearer. Lift it just a little. There."

He rubbed his hands.

"You see, that is better there. I have been wanting to move that for a long time. But I needed a man."

"Yes," said the man.

And he gently rubbed his hands, then he ran his fingers through his hair.

He had walked the fifteen kilometers to get here and he was white with dust to his waist. A bed had been set up

for him in the loft, between two walls of hay; but a real
bed with springs, mattress, those good, heavy sheets from
the wardrobe and then the blue spread with the bluebells
on it.

Madame Massot showed him up.

"Look out, there is the ladder."

"Thank you."

She raised the trap door.

"You have to push it hard, the hay makes it swing back."

"Thank you."

I could hear them walking overhead in the loft, and the
man saying, "You ought not to have gone to so much
trouble."

Massot was smoking his pipe. Madame Massot came
down.

"He's a polite one, he is," she said.

"I heard you," said Massot. "As far as politeness goes,
he is that, but that does not bother me. The rest smells
worse."

"What rest?" said Madame Massot.

"That's so," said Massot, "you have only one eye."

With the stem of his pipe he pointed to the heavy bread
trough they had moved.

"That," he said.

Now the trough was too near the cupboard; the doors
could not be opened wide.

"When one is good for something, one is happy," said
Massot; "when one is useless, one is in the way."

"It isn't convenient where it is now," said Madame
Massot.

"No, but that is my way of being polite. Some other day, I'll say I've changed my mind and we'll put it back. It will do twice."

Usually I fell asleep as a stone drops into the water. That night there were many new crickets in the ashes, and a crazy wasp was still flying about in the honeysuckle in spite of the darkness. It seemed to me that there was some secret between my father and Massot regarding the dark man. I had seen him only two Saturdays in town and then my father had said to the shepherd, "You come in and tell him."

And at eleven o'clock, Massot came in and said, "Well, is the lesson coming on all right?"

"It looks like it," my father had said.

The dark man was holding the book in his hands and the words "magnificent ewes" were still on his lips. (He was reading about all that wild dance of Ulysses and the Cyclops in a round, mellow voice that deepened into sparkling echoes on the word "cavern," that flowed and dripped in milk and wine and swept like the wind and foam over the sails, the oars, the sea.)

"The trouble is," said Massot, "that I am not going to be able to bring him to you on Saturday. I have ewes in salt. I have some that have lambed. I have some about to lamb. That makes three lots. I'd like the boy to look after the ones with lambs for me. They are calmed, their behinds still ache. They think of nothing but nursing their lambs, lying down, sighing like the grass. And they are easy to manage. I'd like to give him this job."

"Ah!" said my father.

"Yes," said Massot.

And so the dark man had come into this good country home. The whole hill could be heard purring, brushing the village with its foxes, its buzzards, its screech owls, its hoot owls, its weasels, its boars, and its rats that hunted the little frogs beneath the bushes. The moon quivered in the darkness like a reflection in a fountain.

We were steadily moving closer to the sun.

The days received heavy blasts of heat that spattered everything with dust to the very heavens. Under the gray shade of the thyme, exhausted larks crouched with eyes closed, their feathers fluffed out, panting from their flight high up in the sky. All day long beneath the sun's fire they sprang like sparks, fused, whistling, to the bed of the blue sky where there still flowed a slender thread of coolness. Their sparkle vanished and they fell back, gray and weary. The magpies and crows kept watch near the wells. As soon as they heard the creak of the chain, they appeared. They would call to the woman who was drawing water. They came to drink at the puddles of water. They would suddenly take flight. A fox was coming out of the brush, running head down toward the bucket. He saw the woman, leaped backward and returned to the hills. He barked up at the sun. The nights were illumined with the bluish reflection of the earth. Daylight lingered on the horizon. Only in the middle of the sky was there night, a gray night, crackling, split with long, silent flashes of lightning. We were steadily moving closer to the sun.

The women talked together a little in the morning.

There were no men in the village now. The women took their pitchers, they went to the wells. After that there was silence, and one could hear the roar of the baker's oven and the wooden shovel striking against the stones. People had to step over the sleeping dogs. Every Monday morning the church was cleaned. The great doors were opened and two women began to polish the floor with chamois skins. As soon as the church was opened, the old men came to sit in the cool shade filled with busy sounds. They would sit there smoking their pipes and spitting between their feet.

The clock in the belfry alone was alive, just enough to say, "Closer, closer, noon, noon."

Everyone was conscious of it. They recognized the fact by the silence.

It was hard to eat. The wasps slept with outspread wings, borne aloft by the sticky waves of heat like seeds.

About four o'clock, the men returned from the fields. It took a moment to recognize them. They made straight for the tobacco shop. They would set their spades outside the door, or they would cry "Whoa!" to the horse. They would stop the roller in the middle of the street and go in to get fresh tobacco. You must never carry tobacco in your pocket. It would be like coffee grounds.

Lunch was always ready at one end of the table. The man would come and he would drink. After that, he would take half of a cheese, a slice of bread, and begin to munch, elbows on knees, back rounded, eyes on the ground, gradually regaining life in the shade.

"Closer," said the belfry. "Seven o'clock. The sun does not want to set. Tomorrow it will be closer."

The man said nothing. He only munched, looking at his feet and hands.

The sun was dropping behind the hill. Then in the silence rose the sound of the earth whirling dizzily toward the fire.

The curé passed so quickly that one had time to catch only a glimpse of his cassock and the swiftly bent sandal.

"Where's he going?"

Fat Berthe ran by. A door began to bang. Men walked past. They had laid Bernard on a ladder, and four of them were carrying him. Bernard's head had slipped through two of the rungs and was hanging, bobbing up and down, and purple in color. His tongue was protruding and frothing.

"No one must go out now in the middle of the day."

"Closer," said the belfry.

They got the barns ready. They went at night to gather heather to make brooms and they began to sweep the loft floors.

Jerome Barrière leveled his barn floor with a great flat stone that had for a handle the trunk of a small oak. He packed the soil down. He wanted neither hollows nor cracks before emptying his grain out. Massot sharpened his scythes with a hammer. Martial sharpened his sickles on a stone. César filed the teeth of his mowing machine. Turcan turned his grindstone. As it was slightly lopsided the sandstone wheel also thumped in the stable. On the one hand there were these hammer blows, these grinding sounds, these dull thuds of a whole village in preparation, and on the other hand, outdoors, the long wailing of the earth as it was being swept toward the sun.

"What is that smell?" said Massot.

He sniffed. In the sticky heat there was a terrible odor, sweet and bitter.

"Something is rotting," said the dark man.

They went out. No one was outdoors.

"It seems to be coming from the stable."

They followed the shade along the walls. Massot opened the door of the sheep fold. It was there.

All the ewes were crowded into one corner. They were all huddled against one another so that the stable seemed deserted, and there in the very middle of the floor lay a dead ewe, rotting. Beside her, her little lamb was still trying to feed at the violet belly.

Toward the beginning of July a mysterious order went from house to house.

The belfry still sang, "Closer, closer."

"Do we attack tomorrow?" said the men in the houses. "Are you ready?"

The women replied, "Yes, we are ready."

"Then, it's tomorrow?"

No. The next day a storm swept up from the sea. At dawn it was already there, having passed over the plateau. From the east and the south it blew dark and damp like a cave; only a tiny blue window lighted the earth from the north, and toward it fled a whole family of falcons. The storm advanced. It rose higher, grew blacker, making no sound; on the contrary, it stifled all sounds, it laid a hush over the world.

César stepped out into the middle of the square. He looked to the right and to the left and he drank in the air. His shirt sleeves were rolled up so you could see his big brown bare arms covered with hair tightly curled by the sun. He shook his fist at the sky.

"You good-for-nothing," he said, his thick lips protruding in disgust.

"Come in, César," cried his wife.

He walked slowly back to his house. From the door he looked once more at the sky. He was talking to himself, mouthing the silent words like bubbles. He shut his door.

A flock of titmice took shelter in the belfry. The nightjars flew under the ridgepoles for shelter. They dug their claws into the plaster of the wall and let their wings hang like iris leaves. Marie Turcan's goat came home by itself. It had torn up its stake. It pushed open the stable door with its head and entered. The dogs were curled up under the mantelpieces, their muzzles in the ashes. Nightingales came in beneath the roof of the washing pool. They stayed there a moment in quiet. They were nightingales from the tall hills and they were still in the throes of mating. They paired off, male and female, under the rafters and began to sing softly in their low, deep, somber voices like forest sounds. From time to time they would stop to listen. But the thick silence still reigned.

"Closer," cried the belfry. "Noon!"

Madame Massot lighted the candle: it was impossible to see the bread on the table.

"I'm going to bed," said Massot, closing his clasp-knife. The dark man was washing the dishes. He went to the window as he wiped the plates and he tried to look at the sky through the honeysuckle.

"Don't go out," Madame Massot told me. "You may go to bed, too, if you like."

"Read," said the dark man.

He gave me the *Iliad*.

I went and sat down on the doorsill.

The nightingales in the washing pool were still singing. Now the storm held the whole circle of the heavens.

The whole day passed in silence; the whole night. The following day, the sky was free and clear. The men and women went out to the attack.

I read the *Iliad* amidst the ripened wheat. They were mowing throughout the countryside. The heavy fields rustled like cuirasses. The roads were filled with men with scythes. Shouts rose from the fields where they were calling the women. The women ran through the stubble. They bent down over the sheaves; they lifted them in their arms, and they could be heard groaning or singing. They loaded the carts. The young men lifted the sheaves with their iron forks and slung them up. The carts disappeared down the sunken roads. The horses shook their collars, neighed, pawed the ground. The empty carts returned at a gallop, driven by men standing upright in them as they whipped the animals and held the reins in a firm right hand. In the shadow of the bushes men lay stretched out flat on the ground, their arms limp, their eyes shut; and beside them the abandoned sickles gleamed in the grass.

We were going up to tend the sheep. The hill beloved of these animals was just above the harvest. The dark man lay down in the warm shade of the junipers; I stretched out beside him. We lay there a moment panting and blinking our eyes. The road up the hill with its round stones shone a long time, twisting and sparkling before my closed eyes.

"And the book?"

"Here it is."

He looked into the bag. The *Iliad* was there, stuck to a piece of white cheese.

The battle, the boxing dance where great fists flew like whip cracks, the spears, the swords, the arrows, the sabers, the shouts, the flights and attacks, and the women's dresses floating toward the fallen sheaves. I was in the thick of the *Iliad*.

The man explained in a voice that penetrated deep within me. Since spring, I bore a strange new thing. At first it had been inside me like a slight taste of green and bitter coolness. The young April almond. It had grown and hardened. It was now exactly like an almond, white, firm flesh, always cold in the midst of my warm flesh and every time my body touched this cold almond with its warmth, long liquid shivers swept throughout my being.

I could smell the odor of women. It was a very special odor. Madame Massot did not have it. Aurélie, the baker's wife, did. Anne did not have the odor, or sometimes only when she did not look at me with her deep, milky eyes. Then she smelled like the rest. And it was at such times that I put out my finger to touch her lips. She looked at me and it was gone, no odor. I would ask, "Did I hurt you?"

"How?"

I did not dare to say.

Marguérite had the odor. She smelled the strongest. She was bigger than I, and bare armed. She perspired as she ran. Then we would hide in the straw. There were three separate odors: the straw, the perspiration, and then the odor. I smelled all three and I wanted to say, "Let's lie down."

We would lie down. Marguérite would hug me tight. We entwined our limbs and lay thus suffering from a dull burning for which we knew no healing oil. The voice of the dark man had the same quality for me as the odor of women. It penetrated me to the almond. He had a special skill in reading—I know today what it was—he entered sensually into the text. He had such a feeling for the form, the color, the weight of words, that his voice impressed me, not like a sound, but like some mysterious life that was being created before my eyes. I could shut my eyes, the voice would penetrate me. It was within me that Antilochus cast the spear. It was within me that Achilles stamped back and forth in his tent, with the wrath of his heavy tread. It was within me that Patroclus bled. It was within me that the wind of the sea broke over the prows.

I know that I am a sensualist.

If I have such love for the memory of my father, if I can never separate myself from his image, if time cannot cut the thread, it is because in the experiences of every single day I realize all that he has done for me. He was the first to recognize my sensuousness. He was the first to see, with his gray eyes, that sensuousness that made me touch a wall and imagine the roughness like porous skin. That sensuousness that prevented me from learning music, putting a higher price on the intoxication of listening than on the joy of being skilful, that sensuousness that made me like a drop of water pierced by the sun, pierced by the shapes and colors in the world, bearing in truth, like a drop of water, the form, the color, the sound, the sensation, physically in my flesh.

He had taught himself to read and to write. He was not obliged to know how pure sensuousness really is. He had all about him, he saw all about *me*, that slime of spittle, pus, and bloody glair that is usually called sensuality. He was not forced to make the right distinction. And if he had not done so, he could not be blamed. It would have been only natural.

He broke nothing, tore nothing in me, stifled nothing, effaced nothing with his moistened finger. With the prescience of an insect he gave the remedies to the little larva that I was: one day this, the next day that; he weighted me with plants, trees, earth, men, hills, women, grief, goodness, pride, all these as remedies, all these as provision, in prevision of what might be a running sore, but which, thanks to him, became an immense sun within me.

If one has the humility to call upon one's instinct, upon the elemental, there is in sensuousness a kind of cosmic joy.

My primitive nature prevented me from knowing woman early. I knew intuitively that her gestures were beautiful and natural and that nothing in these gestures was forbidden; that the whole round world, from my feet to the stars, and beyond the stars; all, all the fruits of moons and suns, were borne in the branches of clasped arms, of mouth joined to mouth, of bodies pressed close. I understood all the simple beauty of this, and that it was right and good. Everything about it. Everything connected with it. But I also knew that the gestures that were so natural and simple for me were ugly, hypocritical, weighted with a sort of black slime for others.

It sufficed me to be touched by the opaque glance of Anne-the-gentle to no longer smell the odor of women.

"She would think it was ugly."

Elusive Anne, Marguérite who burned me, and the baker's wife with her odor. . . .

The world exists.

The dark man was lying in the grass. With the coming of the summer evening, when all the leaves, gorged and drunk with sunshine, were giving off their fragrance, he was there with his books. He talked first with his voice and his hand to point out forms and life all about me. He passed on to me the conviction that all this was not only an image perceived by our senses, but an existence, a pasture for our senses, something solid and strong which had no need of us for its existence, which had existed before us and would continue to exist after we were gone. A fountain. A fountain beside our road. He who did not drink would thirst eternally. He who drank would have accomplished his work.

The harvest was all about us. In the evening, things were more active, they went faster. César wanted to get done. He went into his wheat: his thighs were like the hub of a wheel; the scythe made almost a full sweep around him.

Massot, with his broad hat and his red-brown shirt, could be seen far off. He had loaded his cart. Madame Massot was holding the horse by the nose and fanning him with a cabbage leaf.

The ewes slept in the thyme. Sometimes, without opening their eyes, they would open their lips, bite a tuft of blossoms and begin to chew from right to left, dripping a little purple foam. The lambs stood up uncertainly on their long legs.

"Hey, stream! You over by the stream!" cried the women from below. They lowered the pitch of their voices so they would carry far over this stubble and the untouched fields.

"Ho, we are coming home!" replied the men. The women piled huge sheaves of wheat on their heads and went off down the white road, their whole bodies tense and erect between the weight of the sheaves and the earth.

The men called to each other from one field to another. Stubborn César was still wheeling in his field of grain. He was there all alone. Only his movement and the little flash of his scythe remained in the gathering darkness. The carts creaked along the roads. I knew them, César's, Massot's, by their sound alone. Girls began to sing. The first smoke rose from the village. Night was gently rustling among the leaves and arousing the owls.

Everything had its weight of blood, of substance, of taste, of odor, of sound.

They were burning dry heather in the fireplaces, because it flames up hotter than slow wood. The smell that came up to our hill was filled with the gestures of women over the soup pot, with the sounds that soup makes when it is on the point of boiling and is seething at the assault of a hot young fire. Shutters slammed against walls. The bedrooms were being opened to the cool air. The housewife listened to the clock. It is still running. We'll wind it tomorrow. Far away in the woods, boxwood swished under the trot of the foxes. The stones of the old wall stirred gently. The big snake must be turning around in his hole, rubbing his neck against the edge of a stone to loosen the old scales. A big mound of ants, glistening and growling like an angry cat, flowed slowly toward its subterranean dwelling. The roots of the trees were resting. There was no wind now; only the evening calm. The roots eased their grip on the rock. The whole hill could be felt curling up, and the trees became more related to the air. One felt that they were a little more defenseless, like creatures at a waterhole. The resin flowed down the pine trunks. The little honey-colored drop, as it emerged from the wound in the bark, hissed slightly like a drop of water falling on a hot iron. What pressed it out was the great force of the evening, a force that touched the very heart of the granite rock; little worms as slender as hairs were called up from deep in the stones, and they began their journey toward the moon, through the sponge of what seemed to be impermeable. The sap came up from the root hairs and pushed through the trees to the very tips of the leaves. It passed between the claws of the roosting birds. The bark of the tree, the scale of the foot, that was all there was between the blood of bird and tree. There were only these barriers of skin between. We were all like sacks of blood one touch-

ing the other. We were the world. I was against the earth
with my whole body, the palms of my hands. The sky was
pressing on my back, it was touching the birds that were
touching the trees; the sap came from the rocks; the big
snake yonder in the wall was rubbing against the stones.
The foxes were touching the earth; the sky was pressing
on their fur. The wind, the birds, the swarming air cur-
rents, the swarming ants in the earth, the villages, the fam-
ilies of trees, the forests, the flocks, we were all pressed,
atom against atom, as in an enormous pomegranate, thick
with our juice.

The baker's wife ran off with the shepherd of Les
Conches. This baker had come from one of the valley
towns to replace the one who had hanged himself. He was
a skinny, redheaded little man. He had tended the breast-
high oven fire too long and he was twisted like green wood.
He always wore sailor jerseys, white with blue stripes. He
could never get one small enough. They were all mansized
with a bulge where the chest ought to be. This fellow had a
hollow at that point and his sweater hung like the loose
skin under his chin. For this reason he had the habit of
tugging at the hem of his sweater and he pulled it down in
front until it hung below his belly.

"You are a pitiful sight," his wife said to him.

She, on the other hand, was always spic and span, with
hair so black that it made a hole in the sky behind her head.
She drew it back tightly, smoothed it with oil on the palm
of her hand, and twisted it into a knot at the nape of her
neck without using hairpins. No matter how much she

shook her head, the knot never came undone. When the
sun struck it, the knot had purple lights in it like a plum.
In the morning she would dip her fingers in the flour and
rub her cheeks. She perfumed herself with violet or lavender. As she sat in front of the shop door, she bent her head
over her lace-making and all the time she was biting her
lips. As soon as she heard a man's steps she moistened her
lips with her tongue, she held them in a moment so they
would be swollen, red, shining, and just as the man passed
her, she would raise her eyes.

It was soon done. Eyes like that could not be left wandering for long.

"Hello, César."

"Hello, Aurélie."

Her voice touched a man in every part of him, from his
head to his feet.

The shepherd was a man as translucent as the day. More
a child than anything else. I knew him well. He could make
whistles out of the seed of any fruit. Once he made a kite
with a newspaper, some bird lime, and two sticks. He had
come to our little encampment.

"Come on up with me," he had said, "we'll fly it."

His sheep were on the north slope where the grass was
green and lush.

"When the wind will bear it, I will let go."

He stood a long time on top of a wall and with arm up-
raised, holding the little bird-like object with two fingers.

The wind came along.

"Let it go," said the dark man.

The shepherd winked. "*I* know the wind."

He released the kite at a moment when everything seemed to be asleep; not a thing was stirring, not even the slenderest leaf tips.

The kite left his fingers and began to glide straight away through the still air without rising or falling.

It went sailing over the threshing floors; the hens bristled as they crouched over their chicks and the roosters cried their warning against the falcon.

It came to earth over beyond the poplars.

"You see, that's the wind," said the shepherd. He tapped his forehead with his finger and began to laugh.

Every Sunday morning he came to get the bread for the farm. He would tie his horse to the church door. He hung the reins over the doorknob and with a twist of his hand he made a knot that could not come untied.

He inspected the saddle. He slapped the horse on his rump.

"If he's in your way, give him a push," he said to the women who wanted to go into the church.

He gave his trousers a hitch and came over to the bakery.

The bread for Les Conches was a forty-pound sack. At first it was always ready in advance, and had only to be loaded on the horse. But Aurélie had all week long to plan, to bite her lips, to sharpen her desire. Now, when the shepherd came, the sack had to be filled.

"You hold one side," she said.

He held one side of the sack, Aurélie held it, too, with one hand, and with the other hand she placed the loaves in the sack. She did not throw them in, she placed them in the bottom of the sack. She stooped down and straightened up with each loaf, and in that way she displayed her breasts more than a hundred times; more than a hundred times she passed her proffered face close to the shepherd's; and there he stood, dazzled by it all and by the pungent female odor that floated before him in the bright Sunday morning light.

"I'll help you."

She had suddenly used the familiar *tu* in addressing him.

"I can load it myself."

Now it was his turn to show off. To come on horseback, he always wore a pair of slim trousers of white duck, tightly fastened at his waist by his leather belt. He wore a shirt of rather stiff white linen of such coarse thread that it seemed starched. He did not button it; it was open like the shell of a ripe almond and within the shepherd's whole body was revealed, slender of waist, broad of shoulder, deep of chest, brown as a loaf and all shaggy with fine black hair as curly as young plantain.

He bent down over the sack. He seized it in his fine strong hands; his arms taut. In one deliberate motion he lifted the weight with the sureness that lay in his shoulders; he gave a gentle twist of his whole magnificent torso, and the sack was on his back.

That was all that was necessary. It said: What I do, I do slowly and well.

Then he went out to his horse. With his two hands he squeezed the sack in the middle to give it a waist and slung it like an almspurse over the saddlebow. He unfastened the reins and while the horse was turning, without using the stirrup, and with a very precise little spring, he leaped into the saddle.

And that was that!

"She didn't take a thing with her," said the baker, "nothing to put around her or anything."

It was a terrible catastrophe. You could walk right into the bakery, which was wide open. The baker exhibited everything. You could even go into the bedroom, back behind the oven. The closet was not disturbed; the chest of drawers was locked. She had left her little key ring on the marble top. It was bright and shining like silver.

"Look. . . ."

He opened the drawers.

"She didn't take any underclothes, nor her knitted shirts."

He fumbled in his wife's bureau drawer with his flour-covered hands. He even looked among the soiled linen. He pulled out one of her slips that smelled like a skunk skin.

"What did you expect?" said the women. "Anyone could see it coming."

"How?" he said.

And he looked at them with his little gray eyes under their red lids.

It was soon learned that Aurélie and the shepherd had gone off to the marshes. There was only one road up into the hills and we kept our sheep in the middle of it, the dark man and I.

They came up to ask us: "You haven't seen Aurélie go by?"

"No."

"Either in the daytime or at night?"

"Neither by day nor by night. In the daytime we do not stir from here. At night, as a matter of fact, we sleep in the path because it is warmer and that particular night we read by lantern light until dawn."

It must have been this light that made the lovers retrace their steps. They must have gone immediately up toward the hills to wait until the light went out. A sort of nest was discovered in the lavender from where we could be watched.

The shepherd knew they couldn't pass that way. On one side was the sheer peak of Crouilles, on the other the treacherous slopes toward Pierrevert.

In the afternoon four youths went up on horseback. One of them went without any great hope to Les Conches to have the haylofts searched. Another went to the station to see if any tickets had been sold. The others galloped, one toward the north, the other toward the south, along the highroad to the next railroad stations. Nobody had bought a ticket in any of the three stations. The fellow who went to Les Conches returned late and drunk as a lord.

He had related the whole story to Monsieur d'Arboise, the master of Les Conches, and then to the ladies. They all went to search the barns. Everybody laughed. Monsieur d'Arboise had told stories of the days when he was captain of the dragoons. That required drinking one bottle after another.

From having galloped thus after a woman, and rubbed elbows with the ladies of Les Conches all afternoon, the boy was flushed with more than wine.

He patted the baker on the shoulder. "I'll find her for you," he said. "I'll bring her back to you, but I'll give her a kiss for you on the way."

The baker stood there under the oil lamp. His was the only face visible because he was smaller than the rest of the people and the faces of the others were in the shadow. There he stood with his pasty cheeks and red eyes gazing off into nothing as he drummed with his fingertips on the cold bread counter.

"Yes, yes," he said.

"With this business," said César as he came away, "you'll see that we are going to lose another baker. Love is all very well, but you've got to think about eating. And now we'll have to go all the way to Sainte-Tulle for our bread. I'm not saying anything, but if she had had a head on her, she would have thought of that."

"Good night. Thank you," said the baker from his door-step.

The next day César and Massot went off to the swamp. They stayed there all day silently wading and rummaging like rats. Finally, toward evening, they stood up on the dike and called in all directions: "Aurélie! Aurélie!"

A flock of geese rose toward the east, wheeled into the setting sun and disappeared in the glow.

César's chief worry was about the bread. What is a village without bread? It's a waste of time and a wearying of beast to go to another village to get it. And there was more to it than that. There would be the flour of this harvest, and where would they carry their flour? With whom would they have their bread account, their stick on which each pound was marked with a notch? If the baker didn't get the better of his grief they would be forced to sell their flour to the broker and then go after their loaves with pennies in their hands.

"When a person gets messed up with love, you see what it can do; where it's going to take us."

For three days the baker did not stir from his oven. The batches rose as usual. César had lent his wife to help in the shop. She was behind the counter. There was no question of shepherd or marshes with *her:* she sat there gloomily chewing her thick moustache, and the exact weight was the exact weight. The fourth day there was no smell of warm bread in the village.

Massot opened the door a little way.

"Well, how's the baking getting on?"

"All right," said the baker.

"Is the oven hot?"

"No."

"Why not?"

"Rest," said the baker. "There's still some of yesterday's bread left."

Then he went out in his slippers, his trousers all twisted, his sweater flapping. He went to the café. He sat down at a zinc-topped table, behind the hedge on the terrace. He rapped on the window:

"One absinthe."

Without that aroma of new-baked bread, and under

the burning noonday sun, the village seemed dead. The baker began to drink, then he rolled a cigarette. He laid the pack of tobacco on the table beside him, near the bottle of Pernod.

There was a slight stirring in the sky coming from the south. Over the roofs from time to time floated that light down that the wind carries along as it blows through the reeds. The clock in the belfry struck the hour. In the square little girls were playing hop-scotch and singing:

> "Eleven o'clock!
> As at each hour,
> The infant Jesus
> Is in my heart.
> May he make it
> His abode. . . ."

Maillefer was at his window repairing watches. He had put up his sign:

MAILLEFER, WATCHMAKER

He ought also have added: Fisherman. Unlimited patience, which is indispensable in seeking the ailment of some tiny wheel with the help of a magnifying glass, was abundant within him. People called him Maillefer-Patience. He would wait an hour, two; a day, two; a month, two. But whatever he waited for, he got.

So they called him, I-wait-I-get, to distinguish him from his brother.

"Which Maillefer?"

"Maillefer-Patience."

They were both patient.

"The I-wait-I-get one."

And so they knew which one was meant.

He was a natural born fisherman. Often, in crossing the marshes, one could see something standing there that looked like a tree trunk. It did not budge. Even in March, when a sudden gust of hail began to ring on the water, Maillefer did not move. He would come home with his baskets full of fish. Once he had a prolonged battle with a pike. Now, when anyone mentioned it, he would pat his paunch.

"He's right here," he would say.

He had thick feverish lips, red and swollen like love apples, and a blood red tongue that never wasted its time in talking. He used it only for eating, and then he made it work, especially if he were eating fish. Sometimes it could be seen emerging from his mouth to lick the drops of gravy on his moustache. He had deliberate hands, slow feet, a gaze that could remain glued to the windowpane like a fly, and a big, hard, bushy head, the exact color of boxwood.

One evening he appeared. "I have seen them," he said.

"Come quick!" said César. And he dragged him to the baker's house.

"I have seen them," repeated Maillefer.

"Where? What is she doing? How is she? Is she thinner? What did she say to you?"

"Patience," said Maillefer.

He went out. He went home. He emptied his fish basket onto the table. The baker, César, Massot, Benoit, and Le

Taulaire, they had all followed him. No one asked a question. They knew there was not any use.

He emptied his fish basket onto the table. There was swamp grass and there were fourteen big fish. He counted them. He turned them over. He examined them. He looked through the grass. He fumbled in his basket. Finally he drew out a tiny steel-blue fish with a yellow head and rust-colored back.

"A *caprille*," he said. "Put it on the grill for me, and do not clean it, is a water thrush."

He turned to the others.

"Well?" he said.

"Well! Tell us!" said César.

He related how, as he was planted in the swamp as usual, and just as he spied his *caprille*—a rare fish, which makes holes through the reeds to go into the hidden reaches, and leaps in the grass like a grasshopper, and travels along the roads like men to reach fresh water—in short, just as he spied this *caprille*, he heard a series of odd little sounds that seemed to come out of the air.

" 'Ducks?' I said to myself. No, not ducks. 'Rails?' I said. It was shrill and it rolled like a rail's call. No, no rails, Catfish? . . ."

"Was she singing?" said the baker.

"Patience," said Maillefer, "you're in a mighty big hurry!"

Yes, he had heard singing. After all, you might say it was singing. There was a deep silence over the whole swamp. No living thing could be in the marshes at this time of the day except the fish, the summer breeze, and the tiny ripples

on the water. Aurélie was singing. Maillefer caught the
caprille with a special twist of his wrist; cast, twist, pull.
Twice, three times, he imitated the motion before the
baker's frantic eyes.

After that, Maillefer moved. The air vibrated to Aurélie's
song. He began to track it as he would the shiver of a
sleeping trout whose belly is being stroked by the roots
of the cress. One step, two; there is no splash under Maillefer's tread, he has the knack of lifting his legs and he knows
how to plant his foot, toe first. The water parts noiselessly
like grease. It takes a long time but it is sure.

First he found a plover's nest. The mother bird was on
the eggs. She did not fly off, she did not so much as move a
feather. She looked at Maillefer and clucked softly. He next
found a herring's hole. The females were in the hole with
their white bellies swollen with eggs, and they illumined
the water like crescent moons.

He walked around the hole without disturbing a single
herring.

Now he could plainly hear the singing, and from time to
time the shepherd, who was saying, "Rélie!"

And after that there was silence. Maillefer stood still.
After a time, the voice began once more and Maillefer continued to advance across the marsh.

"It's an island," he said.

"An island?" said César.

"Yes, an island."

"Where?" said Massot.

"In the middle of the river, just opposite Vinon."

The shepherd had constructed a hut with bundles of

reeds. Aurélie was lying naked in the sun on the stretch of grass.

"Naked?" said the baker.

Maillefer scratched his head. He looked at his dead fish on the table. One was a female pike. She must have struggled against death with every part of her being. On the ridge of her belly, between her belly and the gulf of her tail, her little vent was open and the lamp light illumined the tiny red hole.

"She was drying her clothes," said Maillefer, as if to excuse her.

The baker was all for going at once. It was César, Massot, and the others who prevented him. Nothing could hold him, the water holes, the night, the pitfalls.

"If you go, you'll never come back."

"It's all the same to me."

"What good will it do you?"

"I don't care, I'm going."

"It'll be a miracle if you get back."

"What of it?"

"You don't know where it is."

Finally César said, "Besides, it isn't your place."

Here was a reason. The baker began to weaken in their hands and they arrived at a plan. They would send the curé and the schoolmaster, both of them together. The curé was old, but the schoolmaster was young, and besides he had oiled boots. He could simply carry the curé on his back to the little promontory of solid ground just beyond the dike. From there a voice would carry, especially the curé's voice.

"He is used to talking, he is."

The schoolmaster would go to the hut. But in a way not to offend them. He must make Aurélie understand that it was all very fine . . .

"Love is all very fine," said César, "but people have got to eat."

. . . that it was all very fine but that there was the counter, there was bread to be weighed, flour to be put on account, and then, a man. . . .

In short, César added, looking at the baker, if the schoolmaster could not manage alone, he was to whistle and from back on terra firma the curé would take up the argument. By raising his voice he could do his part without wetting his feet.

The next day, the curé and the schoolmaster set out on one horse.

At nightfall the schoolmaster returned. Everybody was enjoying the cool air from the doorways.

"Go indoors," he said, "and shut everything. In the first place, it is ten o'clock, and whether it is early or late, you have had enough fresh air. And besides, the curé is down there at the stone cross with Aurélie. She won't come back as long as there is anyone in the street. The curé took nothing to put around him. It is getting cold out there, and besides he got wet. I am going to get into some dry clothes. Go along, go inside and shut your doors."

Toward midnight, the baker knocked at Madame Massot's door.

"You don't happen to have a little four-flower tea, do you?"

"Yes, I do. I'll be right down."

She gave him the four-flowers. She added a handful of linden.

"Put that in, too," she said; "it will make her sleep."

The rest was all planned behind closed shutters in every house.

Catherine was the first to come, at daybreak. She scuffed her shoes along the ground because her varicose veins made her clumsy. She was to remember that Aurélie did not have varicose veins. Barielle watched his wife, Catherine, from his doorsill. She turned and looked at him before entering the bakery. He stood with his hands behind his back, but it was plain that he was firmly grasping a pick handle.

"Hello, Aurélie."

"Hello, Catherine."

"Give me six kilos."

Aurélie weighed the bread in silence.

"I'll sit down," said Catherine. "My varicose veins hurt. How lucky you are not to have them."

Next came Massot's wife.

"Did you sleep well?"

"Yes."

"That's plain to be seen. Your eyes sparkle like claret."

Next, Alphonsine and Mariette.

"Show us how you make that knot."

"Only, a person has to have hair like yours."

"Feel how heavy it is, Alphonsine!"

"I should say it is! With hair like that you don't need hairpins."

About ten o'clock Aurélie had not yet come to her doorstep. She stayed back in the dim part of the shop. Then César walked past the bakery. He thought he was ready, but he wasn't. He did not stop. He walked around the church, around the washing pool, and once more past the shop. He stopped.

"Oh, Aurélie!"

"Hello, César."

"What are you doing inside there? Come out and get a little air."

She came to the door. Her eyes were all red. She had let down her hair so Alphonsine and Mariette could feel its weight. Her lovely lips drooped as if they had been tasting too many sweets.

"What fine weather we're having!" said César.

"Yes."

They looked up at the sky.

"Just a touch of the sea wind. You ought to come over to our house," said César. "The wife would like to give you a piece of boar meat."

At noon the baker filled his oven with well-seasoned oak fagots. There was no wind. The air was as still as a stone; the black smoke settled back on the village with its aroma of earth, peace, and victory.

On Sunday, at about ten o'clock, the sun was blazing so fiercely that the road, the walls, trees, and the sky began to quiver like white grease. In the midst of all that, the shepherd arrived.

He came at a long ambling gait. He was riding the pie-bald horse that belonged to Monsieur d'Arboise himself. It

had an Arabian saddle that shot flames from every nail. The
shepherd was still barefooted, dressed in his white trousers,
his coarse linen shirt, but in this glare it was perfect. He
leaped from the saddle. He tied the horse to the church
door.

César came out from the shade.

"Where are you going?"

César was already dressed in his Sunday clothes: his
peasant Sunday get-up with the blue woolen sash, a good
shave and a fine twist to his moustache.

"For the bread."

"You tell your master to send someone else."

"Mind your own business."

The shepherd raised his arm and took a step forward.
César seized the shepherd by his shoulder.

For a second they eyed each other. The shepherd gave
his shoulder a jerk. César gripped him more firmly. The
shepherd took one step backward; his shirt was slightly
pulled from his trousers. The shepherd struck first. His fist
grazed César's chin. César put up his broad open hand. He
did not intend to strike but to hold and squeeze. The
shepherd struck him full on the cheek. César recoiled with
closed eyes. The shepherd struck him on the nose. César
lowered his head and leaped forward. He butted his head
into the shepherd's chin. The shepherd's head flew back,
his arms hung limp. César struck with his fist, deliberately
and straight at the shepherd's liver. The shepherd leaned
against the wall; his head rang against the stones. César
struck again at the shepherd's belt. The shepherd opened
his mouth; he shot a fist that passed above César's shoulder.

César stepped back. The shepherd took two or three steps forward, fell to his knees, bowed his head, and lay still on the ground.

They had fought silently, without a shout, in a little space beside the church. Nobody had seen them. César came out alone. He twisted the ends of his moustache, and went and got a drink of absinthe.

The horse was still standing there tied to the church door. The heat was softly and unceasingly moaning in the sky. Then the shepherd emerged, untied the bridle, got into the saddle, still with his accustomed leap, and turned toward Les Conches.

César drank his absinthe as usual, played his game of bezique, won, and went home to dinner.

In the afternoon, when it was time for the dancing to begin, five fellows from Les Conches came galloping up. The shepherd came first, still on his Arabian horse. He got to the café before the others and he reined in short. The horse began to neigh and dance, striking the box hedge with his long tail. The four others came up just behind and as one man, five legs were flung from the saddle. Without stopping to hitch their horses, the five pushed open the door. Inside, everybody was in the midst of a waltz and no one heard the horses gallop up. With a wrench of the arm, the shepherd separated Antoinette from her partner, pushed the man aside, held the woman tightly in his arms and began to waltz. Three others did the same with Marie, José, and Félice, and Costelet's Germaine rose ecstatically from her bench to press tightly against the fourth. The orchestra had seen nothing of all this; it went on playing the

"Blue Danube." For an instant Marius did not realize what
had happened. He saw Antoinette dancing with the shepherd. It is true she was protesting, but he held her close,
and when she recoiled, he pressed forward so that their
bodies were always touching.

"Stop!" yelled Marius.

And Georges and Ivan and Médéric and Clotaire began
pushing everybody to regain their partners. The women
got up on the benches. The orchestra stopped playing.

"What's the matter? Why, it's those Les Conches fellows!"

"Music!" the shepherd shouted.

Marius tried to reach him but everyone crowded in close.

"Music!" cried the shepherd.

He did not release Antoinette.

"Go to bed!" cried Marius.

"With your sister," said the shepherd.

"My sister's churning . . ." said Marius.

The shepherd let go of Antoinette.

"Move aside," he said.

There was immediately a space around him.

"Come here and say that."

Marius stepped forward.

The shepherd still had that clear eye of a man who knows
the wind; only, he also had a look of contempt about his
mouth.

Marius took off his coat.

"What do you want?" he said.

"That," said the shepherd.

And thereupon he raised his arm, putting into it all the

weight of his shoulders, and emitting a panting sound as when a man splits wood. Marius took the blow square on his nostrils. He shook his head. Blood spattered all about him. With his big innocent blue and white eyes he gazed at his bloody hands.

The girls began to scream.

The shepherd struck twice more with all his might, and with well-timed blows, and the second time, he struck him under the chin. Marius opened his arms like one crucified and fell to the floor.

The girls had pushed a bench under the window. They climbed up and jumped out. Antoinette was holding her blood-spattered dress in both hands and was weeping. She raised her dress. She revealed her calves and the lace of her drawers. Marius did not stir; the blood was bubbling out of his nose.

The women were shrieking. One of them ran across the dance floor holding her little boy close to her. She jostled the shepherd.

"Pardon," he said.

He stood there, his arms hanging at his sides. He had not unclenched his fists. He was looking at the prone man. There was a stir among the orchestra. Zani, the trombone player, had stepped down. The youths from Les Conches made a wall in front of the shepherd. Then they, too, began to hit out.

Zani snatched up a beer bottle by the neck but he got a kick in the stomach, and dropping the bottle he doubled up and rolled under the platform. Ivan had grabbed the youngest of the Les Conches boys over by the counter, and he was hammering him with whirling fists. The biggest Les Conches fellow picked up a chair and broke it over Ivan's head. Only the back remained in his hands. Ivan leaned against the counter. The youngest butted him in the chest and he fell like a sack of meal. Under the platform Zani could be heard shouting and kicking the floor. The two other fellows from Les Conches had laid out Barnabé and Georges. The shepherd had two fellows hanging onto him like dogs. He slung one to the ground and crushed his hand with his foot. He twisted the arm of the other man. The one on the ground bit the calf of his leg. The shepherd gave him such a kick in his face that his head rang against the edge of the table. He twisted the arm completely around. He pressed and pressed with all his strength. The other howled and fell. The shepherd crushed first one hand and then the other.

Some of the women ran out into the street. Georges got up.

"The gun! The gun!" he shouted.

"*Haro!*" yelled the big fellow from Les Conches.

In a thrice the five were outside. The horses were waiting, nibbling at the green box hedge. The shepherd made his Arabian rear at the women. They scattered. With a leap he was in the square in front of the bakery. He unfastened from his saddle a huge bouquet of marsh flowers and threw it on the sidewalk in front of the door. Then all five galloped out of the village down the meadow road.

That Sunday night Massot was to come up to take our place so we could change our linen. As he did not come up, we went over the hill to the cliff that looks down over the village. There were so many stars in the heavens that below us it was like pitch. One could discern the village only by the pallor of the houses. After a moment we heard a woman moaning, and then a window lighted up. The moaning was as regular as a song. As we stood there looking and listening, wondering what could have thus darkened and wounded the village, a fire was lighted in the square. It must have been a fire of dried heather for the flames leaped suddenly above the branches of the trees. The huge crouched form of the church was now visible, then, beyond in the background, the flat face of a house which breathed through its open mouth the shadows of men advancing toward the fire. The moaning was louder, for in spite of the crackling of the bonfire and the murmuring of men's voices its singing was still heard.

Another fire was lighted on the threshing floors.

Suddenly a hot wind touched our skin at the back of our necks. We turned our heads. A great light was glowing in the west. Against this reddish light, swirling with long tresses of smoke, the outline of the hills and the mounds of Scotch broom were visible. We had to make a slight detour to reach the other slope. Down in the other valley an enormous fire had been lighted in front of Les Conches. The great body of the house, broad and bare, with every window alight, sent all its glow into the sky. The whinnying of the horses could be heard. The fire down there was so big and so well built of fine slow-burning wood that it dribbled a sort of thick smoke along the ground. We could not see very much, but we heard horses galloping and shots and singing.

"Ha, ho, iron, oh! Ha, ho, iron, oh!"

A light wind flowed through the valley as it did every night and the smoke rose. Then we could see that riders were galloping around the fire. They waved their long sashes. Sometimes one of these horsemen broke from the circle, took a run, and charged at full speed toward the flames. At the edge of the fire, the horse rose like a bird and leaped the flames, with neighing of beast and shouting of man. Tables must have been set up under the trees. Jugs and pitchers gleamed. Ceaselessly the circle of riders turned around the fire and the twinkling of the sparks rose in the night to the stars. High up a little wind wafted the sparks toward the sea.

We turned and looked down over the village. This time all was dark, but the moaning continued through the night.

At the first hour of daylight the dark man said to me, "What was going on last night?"

"I don't know."

My head was filled with the death of Patroclus, and with Briseis, the horse dealer's daughter.

Two riders from the valley appeared over the crest of the hill. We called to the sheep that were in the path. But suddenly the two riders reined in and dismounted.

It was a man and a woman. Not peasants. The man wore soft polished boots that could be heard creaking from a distance. The woman, in spite of her skirts, rode astride, her feet free of the stirrups and her legs bent. They came up to us. It was Monsieur d'Arboise and that Rachel, who, like the other two girls up there, was called Madame d'Arboise.

The gentleman was corpulent to the point of being heavy. His trousers molded his thighs. As he walked he leaned heavily on his legs and bent his knees so that his boots creaked.

"Well," he said.

The woman who was coming along behind him called, "Agénor!"

Her skirt was caught in ten places by a bramble bush that she had tried to step over.

"My dove," said the gentleman. And he turned to free the woman.

One felt him to be heavy and sly, and his "my dove" did not have a very frank sound.

At last they came forward together.

"Do you happen to have any cheese?" asked the lady.

Her head was small and round like a bowling ball, but not fat. Her mouth was wide and curving, and her eyes shadowy. A little veil stopped at the tip of her nose.

"No, Madame," I said, "we just take enough milk for us."

Monsieur d'Arboise wore a hunting jacket which revealed a breadth of shoulder that could support his little paunch. He was chewing a daisy. His lips were as black as coal and slightly glistening. He was close-shaven, with little gray tufts of side whiskers and a beautiful silky moustache as yellow as gold. What struck one was the black mouth, his way of chewing on the daisy, and under the brim of his bowler tilted to the left, his left eye closed and his right eye open.

He continually creaked his boots.

"Have you any milk left?"

"Yes, Madame."

"Ewe milk?"

"Yes, Madame."

"Will you give me some?"

"Yes," said the dark man.

She turned toward me.

"The boy will give it to me," she said. "In your glass," she added, looking me through and through with her violet eyes.

They were violet. That was evident when she came nearer.

"It has got you all excited," said Monsieur d'Arboise.

She looked at him without releasing my hand. She had taken my hand, not the glass.

"You had nothing to complain of last night," she said.

She let go of my hand.

"Give me the milk, sweetheart."

I held out the glass.

"Hold it for me."

She knelt down in the grass, for she was taller than I.

Her woman's odor was strong. Beneath her coat she wore a little blouse of thin silk, transparent and tinted by her breast underneath.

She opened her mouth. I held the glass to the edge of her lips. She drank the milk, then pressed her lips on the glass to make me lower my hand, and she lapped it with the tip of her tongue pointed like a needle.

She stood up. "Good-by, sweetheart," she said.

She held out her hand. I looked at that hand.

"Kiss it."

I shook my head.

"Jealous?" she said. "That will keep you company. Come, Baron."

They were both laughing as they went back to their horses. They mounted. She gripped the horse with her bare thighs.

Monsieur d'Arboise wanted to go down to the village.

"Let's go see if he is dead." And he started forward.

She cried, "No! I tell you no, now!"

She galloped toward the valley. The man wheeled and followed her.

She had left a great daub of red on the edge of my glass.

CHAPTER VIII

THE DAY came when I was to return to school. My father had written: "I shall come for him on Saturday."

It was the end of the vintage. The ewes, now healed, were ready for the rams. Restless and longing, they called sadly toward the village. Massot came to tell us to bring them down. By this time the lambs had good legs; they bounded ahead of us like spray on the water. The ewes followed.

"They are all in heat," Massot had said. "We'll put them in the stable by the fig tree or else my rams will kill themselves."

With their thick muddy wool they flowed down from the hill, without a halt, without touching their lips to the thyme or the lush tufts of periwinkles; they were bleating toward the stables. And we, the dark man and I, we rolled along behind the flock like trees uprooted: he like an old oak, I like a little poplar. The hill had become our dwelling place.

The village smelled of new wine casks and crushed wood.

It did not smell of wine, it smelled of the dregs of wine, the sediment of the vats. It was the end of the vintage. In huge plank stays, the already crushed grapes were crushed again. They tried to force trickles of wine from them. There was a long sticky bar of wood, and at the word, eight strong hands grasped the bar. Then Mérope sang out. The hands contracted as they gripped the wood, and the strength of the men rose in their arms like two great iron bubbles. Thighs were thrown backward, legs trembled, the bar creaked, the press uttered its cry of birth pangs, its belly sputtered a red foam, and a tiny stream of wine fell into the vat.

This wine lay black and curdled in the bottom of the vat. It did not stir. It was smooth and shining and the sun was reflected in it. In the glass it was heavy, flecked with little rainbows and it seared the throat with its taste of sap and green boughs.

After every tenth effort the men with the bar took a drink. They did not wipe their mouths. When their hands rested they were immediately covered with flies like the hands of the dead.

Anne wore a broad hat of plaited straw. It shaded the whole upper half of her face: the two fires of her eyes and her forehead. She was invisible save for her hard little chin, slightly yellow like old sheep bones. She had discovered some secret fig trees where she played "house in the sky" all by herself. I looked everywhere through the groves for her. I called her. She did not answer, and the fig leaves were too thick: she was completely hidden among them. I lay in wait for her. As soon as a tree stirred ever so slightly, I approached step by step, with fox-like tread. I thrust my head among the branches. I looked. It was only pigeons eating the figs or long green garter snakes twining about the supple branches of the fig tree.

Evening came. The village was groaning with its three presses. As the wind blew our way we could hear Mérope's voice singing his songs for the crushers.

"Anne!" I called. "Anne!"

A pigeon took flight; a snake dropped into the grass; the forest of the fig tree did not budge. I, too, turned into stone. It was a contest of silence. My heart was too tender. The night touched it. The wind took it gently in its two warm hands; the odors of wild mignonette caressed it. It was like a trembling lamb beneath all that. I forced myself to be silent and to stand without stirring like those great trees of solid green that braved the night wind with their broad flat leaves. I knew that Anne climbed the trees barefooted. I knew that up there on the branch where she was sitting she had taken off her broad hat and that she would smooth her hair with the palm of her hand. But my heart was all atremble. I could never wait long enough or be cunning enough to win the good victory.

I called, "Anne!"

She knew that I was there with my tender heart like that of a bird. Why lie? Why make her believe that I am stronger than she in the games that I have invented?

"Anne!"

The earth had been sorely stricken by the summer and by man. The blood-like wine stained the plain, the hills, the village, the roads. The ditches were like wounds with the dregs of the casks. The battle had begun back there at the beginning of the summer, just after the storm that had showered us with birds, that had slung handfuls of birds into our windows and drowned nightingales in the washing pool. After that, the men had gone out with scythes, the women with binders. They had dragged the ripened hay to the cavernous lofts. They had trampled the earth with all the horses, they had crushed it beneath the carts. They had torn shreds of the thick flesh with man's tiny beak and claws, but in the end they had weeded and raked and had obtained a harvest of wheat, lentils, forage, wine. It is true, there had been storms and mighty resistance by the earth, with thunder and lightning and slaughter of trees by the bolts. There had been those hard winds like showers of stones. What difference had that made? It had sown confusion for a day. The people had whipped up the horses and fled to shelter. The next day they were out on the plain once more, raking, harrowing, weeding. And now, with this wine, the earth was at last bleeding all over. On the road banks where the loads of grapes had been dumped, the grass was soft with pulpy mash like a bruise. Down yonder in the valley, the still river bred flies like a dead animal. They slept in the reeds, at the edge of the waters surfeited with the sun, rotting, stagnant and green between the stones like broken branches; they dwelt among the mosses; they blackened the sweet willow boughs; they drifted down the wind. But if the wind came from the village instead of from the hills where the forests were slowly living their peaceful life, if the wind came from the direction where the men had stricken the face of the plain and

where the earth was bleeding wine, the flies rose all together in a cloud. They spoiled the bread and the meat;
they came and sucked the mash, even to the sleepers'
beards, to the hands of the men at the bar, to the corner of
Mérope's mouth. The women flapped their aprons to chase
them away.

Toward evening they flowed with the night into the fig
groves. They alighted on the pigeons; they covered their
feathers like dust, like the blossoms of some black tree
devastated by the wind. They alighted on the long garter
snakes, and the serpents flipped their coils and then glided
into their holes with the sound of sputtering oil.

"Anne!"

There were so many flies, there was so much sugary
wind, there were so many pale gleams in the orchard
foliage, and so much silence that the thought of death came
constantly to my mind.

It was my human need to keep from dying that made me
call, "Anne! Anne!" through the fig grove where the darkness was so thick. And so I began indeed to be a man since
I had such a passion for living. I was no longer of the world
of children but I weighed my weight on the earth and the
wind no longer allowed me to float like the light down of
the maternal bush, but it already pressed upon me with all
its weight to force me into the path.

For the first time, that year, the odor of women reached
me. At that moment the world stopped singing. It made a
long pause so that I might be alone with that woman's odor,
of sweet cinnamon or incense when the church door is
open after vespers. And I was alone with that odor; I had

been completely macerated in it. I was quite soft, quite
supple, a rag rumpled between the hands of the world. I
was ready. Then the song of the earth and waters changed
its register. Every word told me of the importance of blood.
Some beast must have been killed somewhere in the sky,
behind me in my shadow, beyond the sky, quite close to
me, and all that I inhaled was the insipid taste of the butcher
shop with its drawn sheep carcasses. The clouds were
wounded, the hills beaten, their backs broken, their heads
bowed; life no longer had soil of winged sand all springy
and dancing. I had to drag my feet at each step through
hot, thick mud, but it intoxicated me like the scent of the
marshes and of spring.

Toward the end of our stay in the hills, the ewes also had
an odor for me. Sometimes I would get up in the middle of
the night. The dark man was sleeping. Without a lantern I
went to the resting ewes. I would kneel beside them, smell
them. I would sniff at their wool as one sniffs a clod of
earth to see whether in plowing one had put all the ferti-
lizer into it, the salty kind, and the kind without salt. Beneath the wool was the animal odor. It was necessary to
wait a moment to get the unmixed odor of the beast. The
ewe trembled slightly in my hands, like very wet mortar,
ready to be spread. The ewe in her sleep was desiring the
ram and suddenly the creature's odor penetrated me. I
saw the village women: Aurélie filling the shepherd's sack,
those passing down the road, the ones leaning over the
washing pool, those carrying pitchers with their left arms
outstretched, those who rubbed their breasts under their
blouses, those who stood arms akimbo, the girls coming

from a dance smoothing their hair and patting their skirts.
Rachel who left a bit of her lips on the glass from which she
had drunk milk. Anne.

"Anne!"

The ewe trembled in its sleep. Beside it there were other
ewes, then others still, in the rough grass, and I could hear
them breathing. Then, there were all those women, and
sometimes the face of the girl perfumed with musk, the tip
of her fingers when she was tying my tie, Antonine who hid
her ewe odor beneath violet perfume, the two Louisas;
then once more the ewes, then the mares, cows, sows, the
women who passed by in the swift carts, girls on the
mounds of hay, Anne with her lips shining like glow
worms; ruffed doves panting on the ledge of the dovecotes,
wild sows, vixens, bitches, mares; swift visions of dances
with music, girls, mothers, children, all mingled, all kneaded
into one dough, all of this stretched out like a great serpent
that lies dreaming as it develops its eggs.

But I heard the ewe's knees cracking and she jerked herself out of my hands. I returned to wrap myself in my
hooded cloak, by the lantern. There was wool in my
hands.

I was filled with sadness.

That last week was dark and long. Every morning, the
day broke upon a vast hard sky. I could hear it strike and
flow along as it jostled the great golden poplars. There was
no color anywhere save in the dying leaves of the trees.
The mornings were as clear as water and the sun still lay
full upon us all day long. In the evening, clouds pressed

their liquid into the valleys hollowed like vats. In the village the sounds of the wine press rang heavy and dull.

I never saw Anne again. From a mulberry tree near the house I watched for her. I climbed up into the tree. With Anne, everything happened in trees, above the earth, in the swaying of the branches, in the land of the wind and the clouds. From behind the leaves I watched her window. I wore myself out waiting. She did not come out of the house. She was not inside. I went to the orchard, I called, I hunted. I began to pant like a dog on the trail. I looked in the grass to find the glistening track of her step on the lucern or the clover. Surely she was in the orchard. Sometimes I caught a word of that long song that she always sang to herself and that at lovely moments of peace and happiness she allowed to slip between her lips in bubbles. I went toward the sound. I called. I was in urgent need of salve for the sadness in my heart, that sadness like a thirst that burned my body after I saw the great serpent born of the odor of ewes. I was in great need of the milky eyes, the black hair, the still, calm face of Anne the odorless, the cold, silent little girl, the sleeper with open eyes, perched in the trees like a fruit.

"What is the matter with the child?" said Madame Massot. "Look at him."

Massot looked at me.

"He was fine," she went on to say. "He had round cheeks. He had color, and now just when his father is coming for him, look at him, he's peaked."

"He is growing up," said Massot.

She went and got her wine of bitter rinds. She poured it out for me in little coffee cups. She tempted my appetite with anchovy tarts, with sauces of crushed garlic, and wild shallots; she rubbed my head with alcohol.

She said to me, "Go on out into the sun, my dove." And she would watch me go with a sigh.

The burning desire to exist eternally that had given odor to the ewes and made the rams battle was devouring me too. "Anne!"

I was unable to sleep. I listened to time gliding by in the night.

I acquired a sort of pointed and moon-like face, a gray mask of sand and plaster, a dead skin. My cold cheeks had melted, my nose had grown thin, with only a drop of flesh around the nostrils that I could feel swell and stir each time I breathed in. There was no mirror in the Massot's house, but I had learned for some time past to look at myself in the windowpanes. I examined my strange, ecstatic, sad countenance. I ran my fingers over my thick, tufted eyebrows; I touched the violet skin beneath my eyes. My gaze came from beyond my being. It had lost its blue color, its clarity, its freshness. Now it was like thick, wet grass. My mouth was swollen and no matter how tightly I closed my lips, they constantly separated into two little horns of raw flesh.

On Sunday morning Rachel and the Baron arrived on horseback for Mass. Monsieur d'Arboise clapped his hands and the proprietor of the café came out with a glass, a bottle of absinthe, and the carafe. The Baron drank four glasses one after the other; he licked his moustache and dismounted. He sat down on the church steps, took off his riding boots and his socks, and he went in to Mass in his bare feet. Rachel fastened the horses to the iron bar of the washing pool, she dusted her skirt with her riding crop. She stood a few moments outside the church, watching the Mass that was burning there inside, then she went off toward the threshing floors, creaking her little boots of Russian leather.

I had not effaced the trace of her lips from the glass from which she had drunk the milk.

"Here," the dark man said to me, "wash your glass."

He was busy cleaning out our knapsack. He was to set out again alone that very evening with a flock of lambs that Massot wanted to accustom to harsh grass.

I went to the sink and pretended to wash it.

"Wash it clean," said the dark man. "I'm watching you."

I rubbed the red spot. It hurt my fingers. I put the glass in its place on the shelf with the others. Rachel had turned the corner of the street. I would not see Anne again, my father was coming.

"Here," said the dark man, "come and see: my knife, the one with the cork screw, and the can opener. Some thread and needles, my book, the litre bottle, two loaves, the onion, the jar of honey, the awl and the wax-end, the arnica, meat and sausage; my cloak and the staff. . . ."

He looked at me.

"That is all," he said; "you see, there is enough here to live on."

My father arrived about two o'clock in the afternoon, in the boiling sun. He had walked. There was something different about him. I had never seen him red and perspiring beneath his white beard. He had his shirt sleeves rolled up on his pallid arms. He did not come at once into the cool of the kitchen but stayed on the threshold to dry off.

When he did come in, he had become once more my father with amber eyes. He took out his comb and combed his beard. He held the back of his left hand under his beard and combed out the tangles with short strokes. The beard foamed like lather.

He looked at me without any trace of surprise.

"He's getting to be a man," was all he said. "His mother will be sorry, but I am glad it is as it is."

There was no use counting on Rachel any more. I saw her throw her leg over her horse and gallop off toward Les Conches. There was no use counting on Anne; the day was drawing to a close, she must be hiding in some fig tree absorbed in her game of silence.

I had to go.

My father walked in silence until we reached the hills. I followed him. From time to time I would turn around to look back at Corbières. The village lay far below like the heaped up ashes of a great fire. It was white and still smoking here and there. Long flights of swallows floated like wisps of grass in the sky.

As we came out of the Isnard road, at the place where the whole countryside was spread out before us, from the plateaus to the river, my father spoke.

"Son," he said, "look. If a person had faith as big as a grain of pepper, he would only have to say one word and all of these hills would rise up like sheep and march in a flock before us to the sea.

"I have been wanting to talk to you for a long time and

I've been thinking over many things all alone up there in my workroom.

"Now, maybe you will become my companion. What do you say to that?

"I am taking advantage of this descent in the road to tell you first what is the approach to everything. Maybe I'm in a big hurry, eh son? But I see that you are ready to hear this and I think I ought to talk to you now. If I said to you: 'Put your hand into that bush and take the fish that is singing on the branch,' you would say to yourself: 'My father has gone mad; fish do not build nests in the hawthorn!' There is something that is stronger than that. And yet it really exists: hope.

"You see, son, the earth and all, and you are going to see our street. You have grown new eyes. Do not be upset if everything around you looks covered with coal dust. The extraordinary thing, the fish in the hawthorn exists: hope. For, when all is said and done, if one trusts what one sees and hears, one has not much reason for hope. Don't put your trust in reason. It is with that that a man puts the rope around his neck.

"You see, what I was saying just now, about the hills. If you sat down in the grass and began to shout: 'Hills, hills, come, sheep-hills, and follow me to the sea,' I, your father, would say, 'Bravo, son, patience; it won't succeed at first, but keep it up. And when the hills arise, come and tell me.' And one day, the hills would arise and begin to move. With reason, one does not accomplish very much. Perhaps a person could make an imitation mechanical mountain, with a secret button, and by pushing the button the mountain would move. That is possible with reason. But if you came along and said: 'I'm going to plant some trees on this moving mountain,' they would cry out: 'Don't touch anything, you are going to upset the mechanism!'

"With hope one can do anything. And the mountains that one causes to arise are real flesh-and-blood mountains and the trees are at home on them and the streams sleep in beds of granite as clean as golden corn. And the force that makes them move is not a force of wheels and steel springs. It is a force of the heart. Once in motion, that never gets out of order.

"Son, if you live long enough, you will meet men along your road who are followed by flocks of mountains. Men who arrive empty-handed. People scarcely notice that their open hands illumine the darkness like night-lamps. When they do notice them at all. And behold, the mountains arise and follow them. And then all the mechanics of reason bang their fists on the table. They shout: 'For ten years I've been seeking formulæ, for ten years I've been scribbling on paper, for ten years I've been working out arithmetical equations. For ten years I've been seeking the secret button. And this fellow comes along and simply says: "Mountain," and the mountain gets up. Where is there any justice?'

"The justice is right there, son.

"Hope. . . ."

At that moment he began to cough and he leaned against a tree to keep himself from falling. He slid to the grass and sat there a long moment panting like a tired dog. I did not dare to say a word nor to touch him. I realized that he was very ill and that he kept it to himself, that it was his personal affair in which neither my mother nor I had any right. He looked at me to see if I understood this. I understood.

"I'm getting old," he said.

My father no longer had any cages of birds. The nightingale had killed itself. It had worn the bone of its head against the bars, then when it had only a tiny film of bone beneath which the throbbing brain was visible, it awaited nightfall. It looked at the lighted lamp, it opened its wings as if for a great flight and beat its head savagely against its perches.

After that my father opened the chaffinches' cage. They flew away. It was still almost summer at that time. But at the first cold days in September, he saw the little pink chaffinch that he had called Garibaldi come back. Garibaldi walked along the window ledge. He looked into the workroom. At last he flew inside and went and perched on his cage. As my father got up to take him in his hands, he flew away.

There was a great storm that night, a cold storm from the first ice in the mountains.

My father had taken all the cages out of his workroom. He kept only two of them, the nightingale's and Garibaldi's.

"You see," he told me, "he alighted there."

He touched the little iron bars. He passed by the nightingale's cage without looking at it.

The sheep court had grown old. I think it had lost its first youth when it lost the girl scented with musk and the acrobat's little girl. The girl perfumed with musk used to sing sometimes, and then there were the white towels hanging outside her window. That white gave the court courage; one felt there was spirit over yonder, that she could spend all night with the light on, but in the morning she undressed herself to bathe. There was spirit also in the acrobat's house with that little girl who never spoke, never laughed, never wept, who only looked out into the gray court. She seemed to know more about it than anyone.

The Mexican woman still sang "Cover me, cover me, I am cold. . . ." But now she could sometimes be heard talking with a man in Mexican. It was not her husband's voice. Her husband had a little yellowish voice like herring milk. It suited him perfectly. He was tall and thin, dried up, burned to the bone. His skin was blackened by the sun, with golden lights as he turned his face. His whole head was flattened in the fold of his big nose.

The man's voice that was over there answering the Mexican woman rolled, lithe and soft, and at the end of every sentence there was a word that rang dully like a billiard ball touching the edge of the table. The woman did not answer immediately. One felt that during this little silence the last word was moving noiselessly through the woman, following a path that the man had planned.

In listening to them I thought at once of the game of billiards. The voice flowed with the sound of the ivory ball rolling along the felt. There was nothing harsh about it, nor sharp nor shrill. It was all roundness, and felt, and gliding. But, as soon as it began, one felt that it had set out to touch

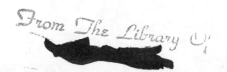

something, that it was rolling along the opposite side but one would hear the dull thud of the last word.

And after that . . . !

The Mexican woman had the voice of a little wild creature of the underbrush, one of those nervous animals, always crouching, who before they die rip the hand of the hunter.

The husband worked in the quarries. He left late in the morning. As soon as the Mexican woman was alone she would open the window and air her mattress. Then she would take her mattress in and she could be heard making her bed. After a moment she began to sing, at first softly, "*Tapa mé, tapa mé,* cover me, cover me," then louder and louder, drumming furiously with her bare feet on the floor, then striking her fist on the table, then crying "*Tapa mé, tapa mé*" with a hoarse growl in her little cat's throat.

Suddenly she stopped. Someone could be heard entering and shutting the door. And the smooth voice began to talk.

In the street, the little bar Au Tonneau, had changed proprietors. At the time the girl perfumed with musk used to go and look in at the window, the Tonneau was kept by an old woman, Mère Montagnier. She had left. She had not gone very far. She had rented a room in the house but she had sold the café. They said that she had come into money. Antonine, who knew everything, told me that one evening the station bus had stopped in front of the café and a lady had alighted.

"She had tight corsets, and guimpe trimming everywhere,

a fluffy white collar that flowed on her bosom and frothed about her neck as if her breasts were spurting milk."

"Be quiet," said my mother, "you're telling him nonsense."

"Look at him," said Antonine. "He is blushing."

"It's your fault," said my mother, "with your talk."

Antonine winked at me.

"Do you want to keep him in a box?"

And she made signs to me that she was going to the coal bin. I went out into the street and came back in by the corridor door. I found Antonine waiting for me, making a great noise with the shovel on purpose.

"Yes," she said, "a lady in a pure white collar, as I told you. A wide skirt, and beneath it little pointed shoes like rats' noses. She took a little boy out of the bus. She had a big sunshade. It was after that that Mère Montagnier sold the café. She stays up there under the roof with the little boy. The lady went away again. And then you know," she said, "the fellow who has the Tonneau now, if you don't mind my saying it, well, he's a man! Ah, yes, he's a man! You'll see!"

He was a tall, slow man who never spoke. He had broad shoulders, a straight figure, and he adjusted over it very close-fitting little jackets, opening in a heart shape over his flat stomach and always buttoned with one button. He wore black-and-white-checked strap trousers. His shoes were polished clear to the edge of the sole and the high heels gleamed like a stem. The cuffs of his white shirts hung below his jacket sleeves. He wore three rings on his left hand. But above his low collar and soft tie of coal-black foulard on which lay the long golden stem of a red flower, spread an immense face of bare sand. The nose was scarcely indicated, like an old worn dune; the rest of the face was a flat, dead desert, where in places the caress of a strange wind flowed in soft curves. In the bed of the mouth the water could only have passed once or twice. The eyelids were always lowered.

He was called Gonzalès. In spite of the October weather which dragged cold soot beneath its clouds through the streets, he opened his door and planted himself on his doorstep, hands in his pockets, but with the little finger exposed to flash his big blue ring, and he let the autumn air caress him. He did not look about him. His eyelids half covered his eyes, and long black lashes hung below them. He took very deep breaths. One could not tell whether he enjoyed the cold wind on his own account or if that motion of his nostrils, that dilation of the openings of his nose, that slight shiver that ran over his cheeks of sand, if that were not the step of the wind on the desert.

After a moment another face came to look at the cold. It appeared beside Gonzalès on a line with his hips. It was impossible to tell whether it was the face of a little girl or a woman, but every time I saw it, the odor of the ewes, the terrible odor, flowed into my mouth like a wine soup. If I returned to the house, Antonine would look at my eyes.

"There," she would say, "he has lost his look of innocence, but it makes his eyes as green as nettles."

That second face was alive like a great hot beast. Long slender eyes drawn out toward the temples, no cheeks, two good round bones below the eyes, a mouth like a laurel leaf, clay-colored skin, stiff, long hair streaming with oil.

"The Redskin," said Antonine. "He brought her back from the Americas."

Antonine knew many things about Gonzalès. At that time, I did not know where she got all those stories nor why she was all moist when she talked about that man, but I often went with her to the coal bin.

He had kept a perfumery shop in some far-off town of the Mexican plateaus, beyond Guadalajara. He had bought silver bars from three mounted revolutionaries. They had kicked on his door and he had come out in the night and had bought the silver bars. One has to be somebody to do that. He had been shot. He had three little holes in his chest, just below the heart, and in his back, a large scar. His father, a former French gendarme, had been a general for two months, then they had hanged him. In his big trunk in his room—and he never let anyone look inside his trunk, the key of which he kept fastened to his watch chain along with a shark's tooth—in his big trunk he kept dried plants, stones of all colors, and wrapped in three thick old newspapers, his father's head no bigger than a fist with all his hair, moustache, skin, eyes, and his gendarme expression; it was unbelievable, and no bigger than a fist.

"It smells like codfish, in that trunk," said Antonine. "You can't tell whether it comes from the plants, the stones, or that dried-up head. It smells like codfish."

As for me, full of my country village, echoing with birds, ewes, and the *Iliad*, I said to myself: "She thinks it smells like codfish, but it must smell of the sea."

The sea and Mexico. The fiery red with which the Mexican country had been smeared on my big atlas. That soft shoulder of blue ocean which beat against the Americas at its slenderest and weakest spot, on that land torn by volcanoes and by great stone gods bristling with teeth and claws, like blocks of quartz.

Every time I opened my atlas I smelled the odor of codfish, and the shriveled head of the gendarme floated on the blue waters of the seas like an island; its long hair, its moustache, its beard spread in medusa-like rays about it.

I could hear the flapping of the Venetian blinds in the little Spanish villages, in the morning air of the Gulf, all white with spray and the pollen of the palm trees.

The step of the heavy half-breed women moved about the fountains in the courts lapped by the shade.

Old Mexican women with elephantine limbs carried baskets of lemons on their cushions of twisted hair.

Young olive-skinned maidens sped toward their bath in the sea in a train of ponies, little donkeys, wolf-hounds, long-haired cats, while the low sirens of the boats floated on the air as they sailed away to the isles.

There were long periods of silence. . . .

These were the noonday hours. I would go up to the loft. Between gusts of wind October still had great golden days. The sun left a little shade only on the wall of the lady of the green eyes. She was smiling that peaceful and knowing smile of those who are at the end of the road, waiting. Upon my return from Corbières I found her just the same with that narrow gleam on her mouth and eye. She must have been silently smiling all the time she had been alone. She knew.

The day was thick and heavy. Doves were singing on the roofs. They had tiny voices of blood and desire. It was the wild hour when the Mexican woman called, "Cover me, cover me," and beat her supplication on the dull drum of the table, making the whole house yonder tremble beneath that regular throbbing. One might think she was treading flat a building site. Over and over. Then she was still. I heard her door open. I laid my atlas on the floor in the sun. It opened of itself to the page of Asia. The land beyond Mexico!

It was a wide, thick, hot country like the blanket on a sick bed, inert from illness and fever.

"Cover me, cover me, for I am cold!"

Sluggish rivers toiled across the plains and through the trees. In the middle lay a vast expanse of mountains and plateaus, grassless steppes, deserts that had drunk the flood, terrible foreheads, dry mouths that were nothing more than arid, mute outlines, dead rivers in vast gray deserts.

Gonzalès!

Gonzalès clad in jungles and swamps. Gonzalès full of tigers beneath his close-fitting coat. Gonzalès who retained in his face of dead steppes the old seeds of ancient devouring trees.

In this picture of Asia, I saw the proprietor of the Tonneau with his silence, his force, his frightful mountain seduction.

> Cover me, cover me, for I am cold,
> Only the blanket of your mule, if you will.
> Your mule's hooded cloak.
> Cover me, cover me, that I may feel a bit of warmth.

Yonder the velvet voice was softly playing its precise game. It could be heard rolling and striking against the supple edges of the woman.

Suddenly, that day, after a moment's silence, the woman began to moan.

It was a soft, sad moan like the cooing of doves, but more rhythmic than the wash of the sea, and it took such impetus from its sadness and its softness, such impetus that it rose in a cry of a beast seizing its prey. It ended in such severe hiccups of laughter that, nostrils aquiver and stifled by the odor of willing ewes, I shut the atlas.

> Strike me over the eyes with your whip,
> Push me along the mountain paths,
> But cover me, cover me, for I am cold.
> Cover me with your body, softer than *la madone*.

One evening I heard Antonine weeping in the coal bin.

"Tonine!" And in the darkness I ran my hand over the good soft face covered with her wet hair.

"That woman," she said, "that woman from his country!"

Sunday. When it rained, it was dark at four o'clock. Then they spread a great cloth on the ironing table and lit the lamp. My father dressed in the warm room. He put on a stiffly starched shirt, he had them tie his little black ribbon tie. Then he said, "Pauline, give me twenty sous." And he went to the café.

We always had boiled beef for supper. It cooked by itself, it gave my mother a rest. She would sit down under the lamp and spell out under her breath the serial in the newspaper. The shadow that her head made annoyed her and she would move her head from left to right to let the light fall on the little lines of close print. Sometimes she would look up over her glasses toward the door or the walls and softly repeat some succulent words:

"The Marquise kisses her lover. . . . Her mother's cross! . . ."

The door of the Tonneau opened. Each time it caused a cluster of sheep bells to tinkle. Gonzalès liked to be notified when anyone entered his place.

This time it was he who came out. It was indeed like him. He made only the shrill little bell sound. Nevertheless his café seemed to be full of people. I had heard the big voice of the spectacle vendor. He was singing inside there. Gonzalès had just come out. He must have put the little Red Indian behind the counter. I could hear people walking in the rain and the drops falling on a leather jacket.

"Pauline, are you there?"

Our door was pushed ajar. It was Césarie.

"Yes," said my mother. "Well, how were vespers?"

"They were long," said Césarie coming in. "I thought he'd never finish his sermon. He did not know what he was saying."

She put her umbrella by the door. She remained standing. She passed her little wrinkled hand over her forehead.

"Sit down," said my mother. "And your sister?"

"I came to wait for her."

She must have run. Her white hair was escaping from beneath her cap.

"He has just gone out," said Césarie. "Now he is with her."

My mother folded her newspaper. "And you stay here?" she said.

"What do you want me to do?" Césarie smoothed her knees.

"*I* would go and get her," said my mother. "I would say, 'Good evening.' I would not even look at him. I would take Clara by the arm and I would say, 'Come, let's go home.' And if he said anything to me, I would say to him, 'Aren't you ashamed of yourself?'"

"He is not ashamed," said Césarie.

"Well, how long has this been going on?" said my mother.

"For three days."

"And then? It is raining, where are they?"

"In Arnaud's stable," said Césarie. "It is always open. All you have to do is push the door and inside it is full of hay."

I had seen Décidément and Madame-la-Reine again. Décidément had grown stout and blue. He seemed to be fed by an interior sky and his skin was colored with a heavy, stormy, sluggish blood like mud. His thoughts moved much more quickly than his body; they went flying ahead and left him motionless, unseeing and without gestures, abandoned on the earth with his color of threatening cloud. Then his thoughts would return.

"Well?" he would say.

He seemed to be asking: "What has been happening down here while I was gone?"

I met Madame-la-Reine on the street corner.

"Come along," he said to me.

When we reached his door he listened up the stairs.

"No, nobody. Let's go up."

He crackled more than ever, but now he made a new sound. His right knee creaked like dry leather.

He had me come in, drew out the carpet, and sat down upon it beside me.

"Listen," he said.

He took out his flute and slowly played in the dark a long phrase full of soft winds. The clouds were scurrying across the hills like runaway horses.

"No more," he said, "he might come back. So I have made haste to play it for you. The end is even more liquid."

He nodded his head toward Décidément's vacant mattress.

"*He* composed that. He mustn't find us here," he said. "He will know that I have played it for you. Where are you going now?"

It was six o'clock in the evening. I said that I could go with him for an hour.

"Come, then."

"Where?" I asked as we went down the stairs.

"To the Tonneau," said Madame-la-Reine.

Décidément was there. His head was leaning heavily on his hands. He watched us approach him. His glance was walking along with us. It seemed to be on the floor.

Madame-la-Reine touched him on the shoulder. "How are you, old man?"

"All right."

"You've drunk your infusion?"

"Yes."

"Your stomach?"

"Better."

Décidément looked at me with his milky eyes. In spite of everything, it seemed to me that he really saw my face and the change in me: my broader but slimmer shoulders, the slenderness of my wrists, that flowering despair that was slowly eating away the branches of my blood.

"You have grown," he said.

It was the first time he had used the familiar *tu* in speaking to me. His voice was full of surprise. It was the same voice he always had, but more male, with a cavernous gravity, a mountain sound, a harsh tone like the wind on the plateaus. He turned toward Madame-la-Reine.

"Have you noticed?" he said pointing to me. "He has made more bone than fat."

There was a great deal of noise in the café. I had difficulty in hearing what Décidément was saying. They were playing *Mora* and the spectacle vendor was shouting "Four!" like a marble saw.

Madame-la-Reine leaned over the table. "You're better," he said. "You feel better, don't you?"

"Yes," said Décidément, "but there is too much noise in here. Let's get out."

Outside, he turned the corner and then he sat down on the sidewalk. It was evident that he was breathing with difficulty. There was surely a wide gulf between his mind and the physical exertion of his body.

"Go and get the bed ready," he said to Madame-la-Reine. "I'll stay here with the little one."

Madame-la-Reine looked at him. He softly rubbed his hands together; but as always when he touched delicate things, his hands did not crackle. He went off without making a sound.

"You don't mind if I call you 'little one'?" he said.

"No, Fountain."

I had called him "Fountain" one winter evening last year when he had played Haydn's "The Clock," and since then it was the word for tender moments when I desired to help him gently.

He sat panting awhile.

"You see," he said, "to me it is like a great fair near a river."

"What, Fountain?"

"Life, little one. You see, it is full of stalls and lotteries where they sell chickens and chances to shoot at the egg, and wheels that give prizes, pigeons, and fires where they fry fritters. It is white with stalls all around me. On one side is the way to the dance hall. Some of the men take little steps to keep with the girls they have on their arms. They buy hard candies. Someone says, 'Wait, you'll see.'

She waits. You take a gun. You pay five sous. They load the gun with a little lead bullet. You shoot. You hit the egg. 'Did you see?' She laughs, and then it is she who puts her hand in yours. Oh! That's not all! You have no idea what there is in a fair by the river."

He stopped to get his breath. He turned up his coat collar.

"Are you cold?"

"No. It is easy, you know, to hit an egg. You aren't standing far away. But the egg falls just the same. That shows your skill. You never try to shoot eggs at more than five paces and it works every time. And they say, 'That fellow is clever.' "

He was trembling.

"You ought to get up, Fountain," I said. "We could go home."

"It's worse than that," he said. "We haven't seen each other for a long time and things have happened. I can't get up by myself any more, little one. I have to wait for La-Reine. He will take hold of my arm."

He seemed to feel the cold chiefly in his back. I put my hand on it. With my hand I warmed the cold of his coat. He looked at me a long time without saying anything. When one place was warm, I moved my hand to another.

"Well, what can I do about it?" he said, keeping his eyes fixed on me. "What can I do about it? I, the river, in this fair along my banks? If I stand up and go to pick up a gun with my hands of water and try to hit an egg, the man comes along and says to me, 'Put that down, you'll rust it.' And then my water finger on the trigger and my water shoulder against the butt! A river can't shoot a gun. I can't see at five paces. You understand, little one, I have aimed at the distant sea egg. The sea egg that was far beyond the mountains, far, far away. I knew that I would have to push my head through thorns and rocky valleys. That is not difficult for a river. And here is the fair on my banks. You understand, little one, to aim at the sea!"

He began to shiver.

"At five paces," he said, "at five paces . . ."

We were alone in the street. I heard Madame-la-Reine coming back.

". . . aim at the sea. . . ."

He touched his friend's forehead with that silent hand he had for holding his flute.

"He has fever. He is having another attack. Come," he said.

He took him under the arms and raised him gently to his feet. He used his heart more than his strength, and that is perhaps why he no longer crackled but his whole body was silent and alert.

I wanted to help.

"No," said Madame-la-Reine. "Leave us. Go back home."

Décidément's head lay on his shoulder.

"To aim at the sea, little one, do you understand?"

His helpless arms hung at his sides.

"Come, brother," said Madame-la-Reine.

And he dragged him down the dark street.

The rain has polished the bare branches of the trees. Winter has come. The nights are dead. There are no stars, no sounds, no wind. Nothing but the freezing cold. The town, lying in the misty hollow, has lighted all its fires. It sweats smoke through every wall. The smoke oozes between the tiles of the roofs and rests drowsily upon them, thick and heavy. Now winter has really come. There is nothing but the cold: no trees, nor hills, nor roads, nor town, nor sky. Nothing. One can think of nothing but the cold. Every morning some men go out of the town and stand by the roadside, waiting. They are still trying to earn a little something. Sometimes a person needs a helping hand to get a fallen horse to his feet, to bring in the wood, carry coal, earn twenty sous. The one they called the spectacle vendor is dead. He talked all night long. He could be heard on the other side of the wall. He used to call baked sheep liver, stuffed sardines, love apples, goose fat, "God's bounty."

"Turkey!" he used to say. "Turkey!"

He is dead with all his appetite. He froze on his trestle bed, all doubled up. In order to put him into his coffin he had to be pushed in by force. It was a poorhouse coffin, readymade to a common measure, and he had writhed in dying because of the hardness of his mattress and because he had big muscles for a dead man.

Someone called to my father from down in the court. He opened the window.

"Who is it?"

It was the Mexican woman. She wanted to have a knife sharpened.

"On your stone," she said.

"Throw it up," said my father.

She threw the knife up to us. She had wrapped it in a white napkin.

It was a big, broad, sensitive knife, slightly curved at the tip; the blade was as flexible as an iris leaf.

My father spat on the stone, then he began to run the knife over it. He was very careful with the edge of the curved tip. He tried the point on his thumb.

"You mustn't press too hard," he said.

He wrapped the knife in the napkin and threw it down to the Mexican woman.

"Take care," he said, "don't press on it. It would pierce an ox as easily as water."

"I've the devil in my right fist," she said.

People worked less and less. There was no more work for masons or for quarrymen or for tinners or painters. The rich lived within their houses without going out. There had still been a little work for wood choppers. Now that was finished. Winter deepened day by day.

Mère Montagnier died. Before finally getting into her bed, she had had the time to dress the little boy who lived with her in his Sunday clothes. He had a royal blue velvet blouse and a wide lace collar. He went and called the neighbors.

"Come," he said. "Granny is sick."

Pointing to the little boy she said softly, "Monsieur Signières."

Then she added, "My daughter will write."

A woman bent over her.

"Say an 'Our Father.'"

She shook her head.

No one had known that Mère Montagnier had a daughter.

"Yes, she has," said my mother. "Her name is Juliette. She went away when she was sixteen. No one had seen her before that. She was in a convent at Mane."

They rummaged all through the room; in the wardrobe and the bureau drawers. There was no address. They found only a letter written on paper with the heading of some café in Marseilles and it promised thirty francs a month for the care of Monsieur Signières.

A Sister from the poorhouse came for the little boy. In his pocket he had a box of rice powder and a powder puff. He powdered his face, looking at himself in the cover of the box, where there was a mirror.

"He has all the gestures," the women said.

They made the motions of shaking the puff before powdering themselves.

He went off at the Sister's heels without a look for anyone.

In searching for the daughter's address they had found a guitar in the wardrobe. There was an inscription on the mother-of-pearl body.

For Juliette to sing to. Her Jean S.

The mason took the guitar and began to run his hands over the strings. He began to play with a kind of pent-up madness. The women were afraid to stir. They were touched to their very depths, in their most secret parts.

They were conscious of their longing and their weakness. One of them gently sat on the edge of the bed, beside Mère Montagnier. The mason curled his lips, showing his clenched teeth. With his music he was saying that no one was fooled but knew the full injustice.

At last the women cried, "Get out, good-for-nothing. Leave us; we must dress the body."

And one Sunday morning Gonzalès was married. He had paid for a dispensation. He wanted to be married on Sunday. He wanted bells. He wanted music. He was marrying Césarie's sister. Césarie, who knew all this, had gone to the lady organist. Gonzalès had asked Madame-la-Reine to come and play at his wedding. Décidément was too ill.

"Go on," he said. "Ah! go on, little father, I'm all right."

"It will make a few sous," said Madame-la-Reine.

I asked how Gonzalès had managed to speak and say that he wanted flute music.

"He doesn't talk," said Madame-la-Reine, "he makes himself understood."

The news of Gonzalès' marriage had gone the rounds, first in our street, then in the little side streets "under the bells" where the Tonneau was well known. It gradually reached every house in town. It was like the flies. It had come in through the windows, laid its tiny egg in some curtain fold and suddenly the news was there with its vast wings of ocean, Mexico, and fine tillage. Césarie's sister, young Clara, had enough fine tillage in the plain and lovely farms on the hillsides to interest the whole town. She was one of the richest proprietors on the plain. More than that, she had good, firm, well-turned flesh, a round face with lovely eyes, and such a noble bearing that all the mountain boys said of her, "She's a mare."

It must be explained that this was mixed praise. On the farms in the hills the mares are not fat and heavy. As less work is expected of them than fair hope of colts, they are allowed to gallop in the high pastures. They gallop about, they play all day long with thongs of sunshine. They act as if the sun's rays were thongs of a whip. They rest in the shade, then as soon as the sun touches their hide they give a leap. With dilated nostrils they whinny and scatter a foam whiter than narcissus.

Clara was exactly like a mare of the hills. She walked with a sober movement of her big muscular thighs. It was plain that she was naked under her dress in all weathers. She did not need a corset; she never wore one. She had nothing to hold in; it was all held in naturally, exactly as nature had intended. Within her hips she bore a fine nest of new babies, perfectly balanced, warm and clean as the oven of a good baker. But she possessed the eye and the laugh of the mares. Her skull was wedge-shaped like that of the hill mares. Her desire, her need, her law, was to bear children, and as she was naked beneath the commanding hand of the earth, she galloped through meadows with her famished mouth. She frightened the men.

The Mexican woman called to my father, "Mister! Mister cobbler!"

"What does she want?" said my father.

He went and opened the window.

"What do you want?"

"Sharpen my knife, mister."

"Are you there with your knife again? I fixed it fine for you. Do you want to wear it all down?"

"No, but I want it for something special."

She looked at her white knife. She held it straight in front of her eyes.

"What do you want to do with it?" asked my father.

"Stick the pig."

"Which one?"

"Mine."

"You have a pig?"

"Oh! Holy Virgin, yes, I have a pig, Mister Cobbler," she said, "you who do good deeds, sharpen my knife so it will enter as it should so my heart's pigeon will not suffer."

"Come on, give me the knife," said my father.

This time she folded it in two napkins and threw the bundle with such skill that it came right through the window.

"What can she be up to?" said my father, looking at the blade that was gleaming with oil. "She has greased it like a bayonet."

The news of Gonzalès' marriage had gone round and round before it reached Antonine.

Saturday came. She knew now.

She went to get her iron with slow feet; she was as if frozen. She stood in front of the stove thinking, then she selected an iron and came back to the ironing table. She had a sort of poison in her blood. It had put her ahead of time among the dead where there is no further need of motion. But her whole body was still struggling. She tried to pick things up with her hand. Her eye no longer measured earthly distances. She upset the bowl for the dampening cloth or she burned herself with the iron. She heaved deep sighs like sick people who no longer need to control themselves. In the evening her cheeks began to darken, that paralysis of death descended through her body. By now she could neither move her eyelids nor her mouth. She could scarcely breathe through her nostrils. There she stood, her shoulders rigid, her arms hanging straight, her legs stiff, as if made of iron.

They forced her to drink linden tea. They had to knock the edge of the cup against her teeth two or three times. She drank without knowing whether it was hot or bitter; her mouth was like sand.

"She'll have to be taken home," said my mother.

She gave us a look and walked to the door.

Gonzalès had given a hundred francs to the bell ringer. When he returned from Confession and entered the Tonneau he found around the stove all the idle masons and two or three women who would have braved the devil for the sweet joy of the fire. All these, without buying a drink, had the nerve to warm themselves the livelong day. They were looking forward to seeing the proprietor's face when the curé had finished with him. There was no laughter nor anything. Gonzalès came in, shut the door, went back of his counter at his usual gait, in his usual manner, and he was

the only one smiling, through a great slit where there was
no gleam of teeth but only an ugly-colored mouth.

After the early Sunday Angelus, the bell ringer began
little fantasies. He elaborated his bell strokes with dainty
twists of the wrist. He let the rope run slack, then in the
middle of a swing, he pulled it sharply clear to the ground
and then the bell rang three times and its wail went soaring
off into the sky like a skipping stone over the water. At
the end, he cut the sound twice by hanging on the rope,
and the big bell—the one that was called "The Black Bell"
—emitted two rainbow bubbles that fell slowly into our
court, shaking the walls, then they burst, wetting the town
with a little shivering, golden rain.

Day broke.

It was pink and gray mid-winter weather, so sharp that
the tiniest whip of wind was like a laceration on one's skin.
From early morning, long boat-shaped clouds crossed the
sky. Nothing was moving save that silent navigation: the
clouds dragging their shadows over the gray plain. Finally
they stopped as if in port; the russet prows rocked a little
in an air current and everything began to sleep in the cold.

To announce ten o'clock Mass, there were little dances
and laughter in the ringing, especially such a mad gambol-
ing of the little bell that all the low tones hushed to listen.

It was really today that Gonzalès was to be married. I
looked out of the window. The Mexican woman had
opened her window in spite of the cold. She was brushing
a large shawl. It was half out of the window, half inside.
The part that hung over the wall was covered with big
golden birds and red flowers.

She was singing, "Cover me, cover me, for I am cold," very softly, without any heart, and she was shivering like an orphan.

Inside the room I saw the long, thin, yellow face of the husband moving about. He said two or three words to her. She pulled in the shawl, shut the window, and they began to argue. They could be seen through the pane; she was shaking her big shawl covered with red flowers and birds.

In order to get this Sunday wedding into his morning, the curé had slightly shortened the ten o'clock Mass and moved back that of the eleven-thirty. Between the two there was a little space, enough to have the organ play.

Upon coming out from the first Mass, people said to each other:

"Why, it is very early today."

"It's Clara's wedding."

"Ah! Why, yes! . . ."

And they all began to wait around.

All the great ladies were there with their jackets edged with fur, their toques, and their high boots; heiresses with their long woolen cloaks, their Tyrolean felts perched on great waves of hair; the little employees of the workshops all spruced up. In short, everything female in town. They stayed there, less to see Gonzalès than Clara. It was very cold. They pretended they had business in the tailor's shop, the watchmaker's, the cheese vendor's, the milliner's; they went in little groups into the shops around the church. There was no one left in the deserted square but the little lady, Sophie Meulan, the young wife of the old notary. She was hatless, a beautiful brown ribbon bow rested on the nape of her milk-white neck. Wrapped in a thick mantle of handsome fox, she stamped softly in her boots, undulating her hips. Her face, blue with dark circles around her big eyes, swayed like the transparent tip of a flame.

For a while she stood there all alone. Then a quick step was heard in the frozen street and the Mexican woman appeared. She had put on her heavy woolen skirt, very tight at the hips and unfurled in twenty billows around her ankles; it swirled about her step like the black mud at the bottom of the sea. The points of her little low shoes twinkled beneath her skirt. She had the bird shawl wrapped tightly about her. She looked at the empty square. She went to the basin of the fountain and broke the ice with her fists. She plunged her hands into the water to her wrists. She looked at Madame Sophie. She came over and stood beside her, close enough to touch her elbow.

"Good day, Madame," she said.

"Good day, Madame," said Madame Sophie.

"We are together," she said.

"Yes," said Madame Sophie.

Everybody was looking at them. The insides of the shop windows were full of faces watching.

The bells began to ring. This time it was for Gonzalès alone, not for Mass or anything else. There was, it is true, this wedding Mass, but the ringer was not thinking about it. He was thinking of the man with the hundred francs.

He was ringing for the man with the hundred francs, with the face of a dead moon, with that velvet voice that he had used when he had asked for all the bells.

The carillon was ending when Antonine softly came into the street. She must have slept all night without undressing. She had become as thin as death. She looked as if she had suddenly made a mad leap to the edge of the dark forest. She saw Madame Sophie and the Mexican woman. She bowed her head and came and stood very quietly beside them.

Gonzalès would not have the closed carriage; he had demanded the open barouche in spite of the cold. As a matter of fact this was not quite certain. Clara had said, "*I* want," but, as Césarie had whispered to my mother, "She has no will any more, she doesn't want anything any more, she only wants him, and it is as if he wanted himself."

The horse could be heard coming up the street, solemnly rapping out his gait on the frozen ground. The barouche was of coarse white willow. It creaked like a basket. All the ladies of the Mass began to come out of the shops.

"What have you there under your shawl?" said Madame Sophie Meulan.

"Nothing," said the Mexican. "The Christ, Madame."

As the barouche reached the square everybody was whispering and nudging each other on the sidewalks. The ladies hid their mouths behind their muffs. The young ladies chewed their little lace handkerchiefs.

"It's just as I told you," whispered the chemist's wife. "Look. Ah! She has passed."

"There, look, she is coming, look. You see, it is true."

"He is sitting beside her!"

Yes, he was sitting beside her. Gonzalès never followed custom, or to be more exact, he had his own custom, broad, flexible harness that could not serve for ordinary men.

"He is holding her arm!"

"Oh! My dear," said the chemist's wife, "call your daughter; there she is over there gaping like a lost soul."

She coughed. "He is holding Clara as if they were in bed," she said.

Yes, Gonzalès was holding Clara in the barouche exactly as if they were in bed. He had put one arm around the woman's shoulder and he was holding her pressed to him.

"Delphine!"

All the young girls' heads turned in unison, their eyes glued to the barouche as it approached the church.

"Delphine!"

"Marie!"

"Jeanne!"

The mothers called.

"Come here!"

"Come along!"

But the young ladies were all in the front row and were following the progress of the barouche like sunflowers drawn to the sun.

"Come here!"

"But what have you got under your shawl?" said Madame Sophie Meulan.

"The Christ, good lady," said the Mexican woman. "The Christ."

The carriage stopped in front of the church. Gonzalès

got out. He still had his face of sand, mouthless and eye-less, but his body was thick and soft, like heavy tree branches; one felt an enormous and gentle strength every time he moved his shoulders, his arms, his legs, his hands, like the fragrant swaying of a wild linden.

He held out his hand to Clara. She leaned upon it and stood up. She stood still in the barouche for a moment to show herself. She was pregnant and had drawn her dress tightly above and below her stomach to make it plainly visible.

For a moment there was silence in the crowd, then a sort of leaping cry, but it ceased. There was Gonzalès beside the barouche, and his presence explained everything.

The people followed them into the church. Madame André who played the organ had been in her place for some time. She knew nothing of what was going on out-side. She was playing a little march, as fresh and clear as for a bird wedding. Gonzalès had taken Clara's arm. They advanced together up the central aisle, already wed, heavy, gorged with marriage. The little Redskin held Clara's white train. She looked all around at the saints and the stained-glass windows. Monsieur le curé came out of the vestry with his altar boys. He went straight up to the altar. Clara and Gonzalès knelt at the two prie-dieus in front of the tabernacle. The Redskin sat cross-legged on the carpet. The priest turned the little key and brought out the mon-strance. The congregation could not manage to seat them-selves quietly in the rows of chairs. The men had kept their hats on. I was beside the shrine of Saint Anthony of Padua. Mère Montagnier's neighbor, the mason who had taken the guitar, was extinguishing the tapers. He blew them out and then put them in his blouse. He tapped the offering box with his finger. Madame André stopped playing the organ and looked over the balustrade.

From the beginning, consecrated bread was being distributed. There were two kinds: first little crusty wafers that were served on a tray, and then real bread cut into pieces and served in a big basket. The mason, who was next to me, watched the basket approaching. He took out of his pocket one of those little bags used to put sesame in. As the boy passed him, he put his hand on his arm to stop him.

"Wait, sonny, wait a moment," he said. "What prudence in this house!"

He began to fill his bag with the broken bread.

"What's the matter?" he said. "Ain't I on the register? Do you think God made me with his cook? You think I ain't legitimate?"

He laughed with his wolf eyes.

"Go 'long, boy, it ain't for the bread, it's for the blessing. If you only knew how I love a blessing!"

The dazed altar boy watched him help himself.

I felt something slink like a dog against my legs. It was Antonine. She was crawling on all fours. She crouched beneath Saint Anthony's statue. She recognized me.

"He is mad," she said. Then she closed her eyes.

I understood that she was speaking of Gonzalès. From where I was, I could see him plainly, him and Clara and the Redskin. He was not doing anything extraordinary. He was quite simply kneeling at his prie-dieu. Only the great arch of his shoulders, his arms, his body, and his bended legs were visible. One had a definite feeling that there was something unusual, something insolent in it all. But look as I would, I saw nothing but Gonzalès, Clara, the church, and the priest who seemed very small to be blessing all that.

I looked for the Mexican woman. She was not sitting with the ladies in the center of the church. Madame Sophie's russet ribbon guided me. They were standing together beside a pillar, near the choir. They were talking very animatedly without looking at each other. I moved toward them.

Madame Sophie's face was very red and I could see that her hands were trembling.

"I tell you to give it to me," she was saying.

"Ah, Madame! Ah, Madame!" chanted the Mexican softly.

She cooed tenderly as if to soothe an infant. Madame Sophie was in a fury and she clenched her fists and trembled.

"Give it to me!"

"Little madame, little, little, little. . . ."

"Give it!"

The Mexican woman began to talk to herself in Spanish and gradually she clenched her teeth and grew savage as her anger rose within her. Her cheeks gleamed like copper.

"Give it, give it, give it!" Madame Sophie repeated tirelessly. "Give it, he won't suspect me, and I'll strike for both of us."

From time to time the little side door creaked and then closed silently. It was our people from "under the bells," the inhabitants of the sheep court, the customers of the Tonneau who were arriving. The fine ladies tried to get out. They were making all sorts of signs to their daughters. The latter neither heard nor saw; they were all together and gazing silently at Gonzalès' mountaineer back, and beneath the white dress, where, as usual, Clara was naked, the bluish shadows.

For some minutes the church was without music. The curé had turned and faced the couple. He advanced toward them, arms courageously outspread. He held the ring in his fingertips.

Then, high up in the organ loft, Madame-la-Reine began to play the flute.

With the first notes I tried to guess: Haydn, Mozart, Bach?

In a terrible silence everyone listened.

After a moment Gonzalès turned his head. He looked up toward the organ, and for the first time, in the middle of his dead face, I saw his eyes. They were tenderly human.

It was over.

Gonzalès took his wife's arm. He passed close to the pillar where we were, Madame Sophie, the Mexican woman, and myself. His back touched the Mexican. She did not stir. She unfolded her arms and something fell to the ground. It was the iris-leaf knife. Madame Sophie stooped down quickly and picked it up. Gonzalès held out his open hand. Madame Sophie gave him the knife.

"Thank you," he said with downcast eyes, and he put it in his pocket.

As he moved away, the Mexican woman slid along the pillar to the ground.

"Mother, mother," she whispered, "I am ill."

I met Madame-la-Reine near the side door of the church.

"What was that you were playing?" I asked. "Whose was it?"

"Nobody's," he said. "Nobody's and everybody's. Those were Mexican songs. Gonzalès sang them to me."

Everybody was pushing to get out. He drew me toward the Virgin's dark little chapel.

"Ah! How lovely it is!" he exclaimed. "What did you see in all that?"

"That all was destroyed," I said.

He seemed to be dreaming, to be looking through me toward the sun.

"Muleteers' songs," he said, "laments, the early plowmen, woodcutters. . . ."

He seized my arm.

"There is one," he went on, "a youth who carries water to the quarrymen in the mountain. He went to fill the skins at the village fountain. His sweetheart said to him: 'Go away with your devil's sweat. My new love is fresh as the lilacs.' He goes into the tavern. He dances with all his might on the wooden floor and begins to shout like a mad-man:

> I trample my heart,
> I leap upon my heart.

"I had told the lady at the organ to go 'boom boom' with her big bass pipe, the low F to make the sound of feet and of that heart spurting beneath the heavy shoes. She did not dare. Do you understand?"

"Yes," I said. "I didn't at first. All is destroyed."

"All," he said, "all that is there. There is nothing left but the clay. But that extends to the mist on the horizons."

And he opened his arms wide to make me understand that the world remained whole after the destruction.

"The mountain that shut out the sky," he said, "is nothing but a rose made of sand. But the tiny watermelon seed is there before my eyes with its mass of roots and its forest of leaves, do you understand?"

He was waving his hands and arms without crackling.

"A slip of ivy there in that pillar," he went on, "and you can make the biggest statue of the Lord. You can make it of marble or granite, and you will see that the ivy will eat its smile and remove the stones of its skull, and you will see that the Lord's brain will be that ivy coiled within his head like a green snake. Let time alone and there will be nothing here but a forest of ivy with just a bit of dust on the leaves.

"I am hungry," he said. "Gonzalès paid me. We'll go buy an anchovy tart. My brother loves them. Come along."

We went out together.

"You understand. Gonzalès belongs to us, so does Clara. She didn't know it. Now she does. There are not a few who are smaller than they realized and who found it out today." And he pointed to the chemist's wife gesticulating amidst her furs.

We bought the hot oil and anchovy tart.

As we went up the stairs he turned to me. "Liberty," he said, "when it approaches the earth, it has a velvet roar like a comet."

He opened the door.

"Brother!" called Madame-la-Reine.

Décidément did not stir. He was looking fixedly at the window.

He was dead.

CHAPTER IX

THE LANDLADY decided to rent Tante Eulalie's apartment. It was up on the third floor opposite my father's workroom. I remembered once having seen this vast dark room. It was a long time after old Eulalie's death and they had taken out all the furniture and tried to fumigate it by burning sulphur. They had opened the door again, I don't know why. The landing was chilled by that open door. I had tried to see in without entering. It was impossible. The darkness had hardened in there during all those years.

It was only toward the middle of the day that a ray of sunlight penetrated the closed shutter, through a knothole, and then from the doorsill I could see the apartment. It was simply one large indistinct room with an alcove. There were no other walls between that and mystery. In the place where, in the old days, the walls of the room must have been, now were nothing but heavy mists inhabited by countless spiders. The alcove yawned in the background like an undersea cavern. It must be the lair of some coiled, sticky monster, all mouth and big eyes.

The landlady decided to rent it because the frost had killed the almonds. She hired by the day a fat woman who was called "the sow," and it was she who reconstructed the walls. Toward evening she went and emptied on the trash heap a great bucketful of spiders.

It was Franchesc Odripano who rented the room. He must have been about sixty years old. He held himself as straight as a yew. He wore on his head a big woolen cap, the visor of which covered his left ear, and over his forehead frothed a magnificent tuft of curly hair, as white as fountain spray. When he took off his cap his forehead was illumined. He still had all his wool-like hair, but on each side of his head above the temples were two beautiful round little mirrors of skin, smooth and polished, and ivory colored, and the light was there. This light came toward you and touched you. One did not see Odripano's eyes, one only knew that they were light; only the two fires of his temples struck your flesh gently like the pale horns of young rams.

He met me on the stairs. He had his cap on.

"My name is Franchesc Odripano," he said.

His mouth took pleasure in saying that name; it made all the necessary motions in pronouncing it and the lips lingered over every letter.

He went to the landlady. He paid six months in advance. He went back up to his room waving the receipt to dry the ink.

"Do you know where a person can buy some lime?"

He got someone to lend him a bucket, a ladder, a big

brush. He daubed the walls. He rubbed the floor with hydrochloric acid. He bought a table of unpainted wood and two chairs.

He had not invited me to come into his room. He left his door open and waited. One day he said to me, "Why don't you come in? Come in."

The walls of the room were now creamy and bluish like beautiful milky depths. There was nothing in the room but a deal table, two chairs, and a large cushion of Venetian leather on which Odripano must have slept.

"My mother was young," he told me, "but I had my two grandfathers, my two grandmothers, and my father was old. It was a house full of old people. In the evening they lighted the lamp. My father's father, who had been a captain of the militia, used to say, 'Let's show our hands.' We sat around the table; my mother went to get a great silver platter and we would all put our hands in this platter. The lamp light stopped at our wrists. We lived on the harbor. But my grandmother had nailed the window with those big iron nails that they call at home 'Christ's thorns.' Outside the sailboats flapped their sails. The red lanterns at the tops of the masts looked in at us through the panes. We were not allowed to speak. We let our hands lie in the platter. I was four years old. The captain's hands were cold and dangerous like glass. He powdered them with my mother's rice powder. Every evening a sailor came into our great hall and called, 'Angiolina! Angiolina!'

"The servant went down and was seen no more until

the next day. She had a big cloth pocket under her skirt and when she came home in the morning, she lifted her skirts, held them with her chin, she undid the string of the pocket which was stuffed with vanilla, pepper, and sometimes tobacco.

"My mother had lovely sad eyes. She dressed herself in long gowns, fitted at the waist and ballooning at the hem. She spent a long time beautifying herself in front of her mirror with cosmetics from a little lacquer box. Then she had the right to walk through the rooms. But beforehand, my grandmother went to see if the windows were still nailed tightly and she shot all the bolts. My grandfather Horatius tapped with his cane.

" 'Faster,' he would say.

"My mother walked faster and the silk of her gown began to sing. Then my grandfather Horatius smiled. Sometimes at those moments I would approach my mother to touch her. She, too, wanted to touch me and I could see that she was looking at me without moving her head and her hands were ready. My father threw the cane at my legs. Then my mother wept and my father would say to her, 'I bought you, you and the child together, but you've got to obey. Now, walk.'

"She would begin to walk once more and to smile.

"When she was alone I could hear her saying, 'Death never comes to our house. Why?'

"She said to the servant, 'You *do* leave the door unlocked when you go out, don't you?'

" 'Yes, mistress.'

"She would get up in the middle of the night to go see

if the door was really open. She would look up and down the street.

" 'And that Death,' she would say, 'what can she be about? How long we have been waiting for her here!' "

Every time I left Odripano's room, I had to touch the ground carefully to see whether it was still there under my feet. He always talked to me aloud in his bare room. At first there was only his voice, but after a little, when the air was warmed, the echo of the walls began to play and there were three or four voices mingled. Then, in the background of the discourse, a little drumming began like the drum that makes the bear dance, and it would touch my stomach as if with fingers. Then all was peopled with various voices, broken and reflected echoes, slow sounds that arrived after having bounced against all four walls; then it was a conversation with the inhabitants of the mystery, and the story screamed about Odripano like the whirling of a great flock of birds.

He did not make any gestures. He put his arms on the table and he did not move them after that. Only his hands sometimes came to life, but just to close his fingers like lily buds. I was seated on the other chair. He would look at me.

He seldom went out. He lived on cold things: milk, bread, goat's milk cheese. There were no crumbs in his room, nor any odor, save the odor of whitewash.

My mother asked him, "Don't you sometimes get tired of being in there, Monsieur François?"

"No," he said, "but my name is Franchesc."

"In our house," he told me, "there were five great rooms, one after the other. But the walls of the house had been closed around a vast space and one could gallop horses around what was left empty. My grandfather Horatius lived in the first room. His room smelled of fire and spit. He continually smoked long black cigars that Angiolina stole from the sailors. He had catarrh. He would put his lighted cigar on the furniture and begin to cough and spit beside him, always in the same place until he had made a puddle. During this time the cigar was burning the wood and the hangings. The grandfather would strike it with his big hand. When he had finished coughing, he would light his cigar again and change his seat so he could spit in a fresh spot. But in my mother's room there was the odor of cloth and looking glass. She also had necklaces of great yellow stones. She never wore them; she would amuse herself making them dance in their little caskets and when she did that the dust from all that friction flew about and illumined the whole room. After a moment my mother would shut her eyes and sniff. She said that it smelled like a stone quarry in the Roman hills where she used to ride every morning when she was a girl. My mother's mirrors had an odor, too. I used to stand beside her while she made herself up, and she was always making herself up. When she had finished perfuming herself and coloring her eyes, her lips, her cheeks, she would look at herself and then clean it all off and begin afresh. By dint of all this, there appeared in the corner of her mouth a little living sore, quivering with a drop of blood like the tip of a weasel's nose. She would cover it with rice powder:

it would stay hidden a moment, then it would reappear. She would sit waiting and watching, her puff in her hand, ready. You could see the powder reddening, then a tiny pearl of blood would swell. She would add more powder. In her boxes she had make-up and perfumes. Make-up for each perfume. Thus, sometimes she would color her lips blue, her cheeks green, and perfume herself with violet.

" 'You see,' she said, 'look, a tree is strangling me. It has come up to my neck with its big branches and it is squeezing me and I am going to die. You see, I am already green and my blood is rotting on my lips.'

"Then she would stick out her tongue and I would begin to cry, because when she pretended to choke she would roll her lovely gold eyes, with their white and yellow tints. It was just as when the waves turn over the round stones on the beach and reveal their dirty side. But I was quickly consoled by the fact that her protruding tongue was red, and red was a living color to me. The sailboat anchored in front of our palace had a red lantern at the top of its mast.

"At other times she made a cream-colored base which she mixed in a saucer. She waited until the glaze was dry, then she would try the play of her laughter. The little coating would crack at the wrinkles in her cheeks. She would scale it off with her fingernail and cover the place with softer glaze. She would try again until she had found the limits of her smile. When she succeeded in that she surrounded it with a serene tint of pink marble.

" 'Stand off,' she would say.

"I would stand off and there before me was a porcelain doll. At first it would not stir, then I could see the eyes lighting up like the watch fires of the shepherd in the mountains, then a rustle of snow along the nose, then the mouth would open like an autumn full of grapes and my mother's face in its smile was as lovely as the livelong year. She was so pleased with my joy that I could hear a little snap like the lid of a box falling shut; it was her laugh, her free young girl's laugh that was cracking the enamel. It fell off her cheeks in bits and underneath I could see the dead skin, sunless and dry.

" 'Ah,' my mother would sigh, 'when Death comes to this house, Franchesc, I shall say to her, "Help yourself, help yourself, kind lady"; then we two shall depart with the sailors.'

"There was another odor in my mother's room. It was that of a new whip.

"The door would open. My father came in. He leaned on two canes. He was heavy and tall. He was frozen from his feet to his armpits. I called him 'Monseigneur.' Only his arms, his shoulders, and his countenance already devoured by the moss of age, were free. He would look at my mother. She sat motionless; she crossed her outspread hands on her breast. He would say to me, 'Get out.' "

Franchesc's stories never had any point or ending. They would wander at random like pigeons. They would fly, calling, in all directions, and the house was henceforth inhabited by these screaming tales. They never died. Sometimes they were found long after in some dark corner. There they were waiting, and sometimes they would leap up at one.

Since the arrival of this man, I had not looked into the sheep court more than once or twice. And then, it had not been of my own will, but by the impulsion of a sort of inner reproach. That world of Décidément and Madame-la-Reine, the Mexican woman, the girl perfumed with musk, Death seemed to be slashing out savagely at it all. Madame-la-Reine no longer went out except sometimes in the evening. He had lost his old familiar look and now his face was like some abandoned ruin in mid-forest, far from men, all alone with the plants and the wild creatures. His hair was eating his cheeks; two great roots of blond beard were beginning to loosen the joints of his lips. When he tried to play the flute now, he was obliged to push this hair back with the palm of his hand. Then he would try to set his mouth in its old shape. It was very difficult. One felt that below his head, in the damp cave of his breast, he was full of hair seeds and that it was useless for him to hope: his fate was to be eaten by those animal hairs and to fall slowly in ruins beneath his beard. Moreover, he no longer made any effort and he would spend his days sitting crouched on his carpet. Décidément's violin lying upon his lap, and from time to time he would pick the strings in the rhythm of a slow, slow melody like a long thought.

Once I met him in the street. He pushed me aside with his hand.

"No, no, I haven't time."

The Mexican woman still sang "*Tapa mé*." She had lost all her branches, all her leaves, all her bark, her verdure. She was nothing but a hard, dried-up object. One had the impression that a slow fire was eating her marrow and that she was a seething brasier within, that one day she would suddenly fall to ashes without leaving a trace. At night she would go and wait for men on the street corner. I walked around her once without daring to pass her.

Antonine had gone.

The sheep court smelled of defeat and slavery. In this camp of the vanquished nothing remained but submission and death. It stayed there on its dung. From time to time the butcher would come in and take an animal to the slaughter house.

Even my father. . . .

He was more and more alone. His heart did not help him now. He could still help others, but he had no more aid for himself and there was my father with the others, seeing his city destroyed, his fields burned, and himself forced to set out alone on the highways like the rest.

One evening we were just at the end of our evening meal. We heard someone cry, "Help!"

My father stood up. "Come along," he said.

I came behind him. It was at the wheelwright's house. There was the sound upstairs of a man's heavy breathing as if he were putting all his strength in some weighty task. The cry was not repeated.

"What are you up to?" cried my father opening the door.

The wheelwright was killing his son. The boy was already crucified against the wall, his arms outstretched, his head hanging. A trickle of blood dropped from his lips.

The man had pushed the heavy table against the boy and was crushing his chest. Over by the window the mother was trying to breathe, to keep alive in order to call for help. She could only shake her head as the horses do when they are chasing away the flies.

I did not have time to make a move.

The wheelwright was already in a heap over by the wall. He did not know where the blow had come from. He was panting in his moustaches and looking at his hands. He looked as though he was going to sleep.

I knew that my father was not strong, that he was old, already stricken with the disease of which he was to die.

"Are you crazy?" he said. "Get some water, woman."

"Yes," said the wife.

She did not move. She could not. She was trembling all over.

"Help me," said my father.

I lifted the heavy table away. The wheelwright lay crumbled in a heap, snoring.

"Little fellow," said my father.

He touched the boy's cheeks. He washed him, then he took him by the waist and carried him away without anyone's help.

That night I slept on the bedside mat. I had given my place to the wheelwright's boy. He was moaning feebly.

My father was a long time getting to sleep. I was lying next to his bed. He called me: "Jean!"

I put up my hand to touch him. I met his hand coming down to me.

"I can't explain it," he said in a whisper. "Did you see? I don't understand! I just put my hand on his shoulder and he fell like dust."

Franchesc was not defeated. You had only to look at him. Nevertheless he was one of us.

I often wondered why he belonged to us, in spite of that Monseigneur of a father and that palace on the seashore where the sailboats came to anchor in vain. He had his grace, his cleanliness, and that feeling for walls. He was the only one who had bought whitewash. He loved soft white shirts that billowed like clouds and sometimes in his room he would go barefoot, with lovely, well-shaped feet, relaxed and happy like hands. His hand was long and slender. It began opposite the thumb with the dizzy rise of a sheer little finger like the side of a glacier; two leaps raised it to the summit of the middle finger. There, it seemed, was the inaccessible aerie in the heights, then it descended on the side of the thumb by way of the index finger, and at the edge of it dropped an abyss. Far below in the valley the sides of the thumb took root in the broad palm where three deep rivers swept down the waters of destiny. And in spite of all that, he belonged to us, to the poor and the lost, to those whom, in spite of His goodness, Jesus had had to leave in the net. He belonged to our sheep court. Over him, too, Jesus had stretched His hand and had said, "It is too bad for those; I cannot hold everything; who embraces too much, embraces futilely." He was, like us, outside the arms of God, forgotten of God Himself. He

was not defeated. With ease he bore on his forehead a
magnificent victory.

I found him laughing.

"I saw the confectioner," he said. "He was in front of
his shop. He had made a fortified castle out of praline paste.
It is in his window. He said to me, 'Now, I am going to
melt the whole thing and make the bridge across the
Durance.'"

He grew serious.

"That's the way with pastry," he said.

He continued:

"When my mother made up as the porcelain doll, she
perfumed herself with rose. Each perfume bottle went with
its box of make-up. She had studied it all out and never
made a mistake. As long as she was in front of her mirror,
the world on the other side was inhabited by her reflection.
And that reflection did not always do the same things she
did, but it seemed more alive, more vigorous; it had more
courage. It could not have been beaten with the whip, or
that would have happened only once, and the reflection
would have departed immediately with the sailors, taking
with it its little dream boy. Sometimes the reflection would
open its blouse and one could see beautiful breasts ready for
the adventure, hard and swollen like gallant sails. That
woman opposite was looking at us, but she went away as
soon as my mother got up to get another box of paint. She
faced the world with motions of such grace and strength
that a different perfume from that of my mother's came to
me through the looking glass.

"I had two grandmothers: Madame Horatius and Madame Captain. Madame Horatius nailed the windows shut with the long iron nails. The rest of the time she made bolts. She had a locksmith's shop set up in her room, with a vise and a panoply of files. She had achieved such skill that her bolts slipped into their staples like dream bolts. But under her lace mitts her oily and dirt-stained fingers full of metal shavings were like roots of bronze. She never washed and her bread tasted of metal. Sometimes she would offer me little crumbs of bread broken with her fingertips. I would keep them in my mouth without chewing them, then I would quietly throw them behind my back, since once a splinter of iron had made my lips bleed.

"Madame Captain was in love with love and that is why she was suspicious. She discovered the odor before me, perhaps even before my mother. That is why Death entered the house but chose the most beautiful, the one who longed to be off to the hill of Fiesole.

"You could do anything you wanted with Angiolina. You had only to fasten her to the table leg with scarves. The men would call, 'Angiolina! Angiolina!' from below in our hall.

"The girl would writhe and sometimes drag the big table a few feet.

" 'Vacca,' said my mother. 'You are a cow. They are downstairs calling you. Say that you will bring it.'

"It was plain that the girl had nothing left, neither head, nor body, nothing save her desire.

"My mother undid the scarves.

"One night Angiolina said, 'I will bring it to you.'

" 'Swear,' said my mother.

" 'By the Seven Wounds.'

"Then my mother took me in her arms and she rocked me a long, long time in her young girl's arms and she sang me the song:

> His jersey is striped with blue,
> And he knows the island routes.

"Angiolina came back in the middle of the night. A huge star lighted the window. The cables creaked along the wharf and the lagoon rippled beneath the calm sweep of a sailboat bound for Africa.

" 'Take it quick.' And she gave my mother a handful of little brown seeds.

" 'I could kiss you,' said my mother.

" 'Doesn't that burn you?' asked Angiolina.

" 'No.'

"My mother was daintily holding the handful of seeds.

" 'Would Christ think it is right?'

" 'Yes,' said my mother. 'Kiss me.'

"My mother," he went on, "was the Pope's niece. That night she kissed Angiolina for the handful of seeds. She kissed Angiolina on her mouth, and Angiolina's mouth smelled of rotted boat and dead sailor; it was the sink of the sea world, and all the sailors during their nights on the main thought of Angiolina's mouth but not her kiss.

"The star illumined the two women. The sailboat had passed the cape; we could hear the flapping of its sails. My mother kissed Angiolina with the tenderness of a dove, very gently around her lips and on her lips."

For the first time, Odripano raised his hand and spoke directly to me. He looked at me with his eyes so strangely fixed that at last I saw their color. They were blue, blue like mine.

"Son," he said, "one must be full of forgiveness. One must have more forgiveness in one's body than blood.

"I say this, not for what my mother does, but for what she is going to do."

He became motionless once more, leaning on the deal table. He lowered his eyelids, and while the lights on his forehead glowed like fanned fires, he went on in his voice that was like the sea.

"My mother puts on her black dress. It is a Tyrolean dress laced over the white silk of her breast. It is all adorned with embroidered birds and dancing serpents. But with her fingernail she pulls out the embroidery stitch by stitch. At the end of the day she stands up, she shakes out the threads and this time she is all in black save for the lacings on her breast and heart. She has her calm open countenance, her nostrils ready for the wind, and the wide smile of the knowing gods.

" 'Death is coming, Franchesc. I wrote to her with my blue ink, and my little handwriting that goes slanting down the page, and she has answered: "Count on me."

" 'You must be a good little boy with her for she is going to help us, you and me. *I* will do the honors. I shall say to her, "There is Monseigneur, there is Monsieur Horatius and Monsieur Captain, and there are the women who wish to go with them." She is coming to invite them. She will take them by the hand and lead them to her country. I told her that Monseigneur was not your father, that I was not his wife, and she will not invite us two. We will remain all alone. Then we shall go to the hill of Fiesole to find the one I love, the one I called Saint Francis and who called me Saint Claire. The one of whom I thought when I made you.'

"I asked her if we were not going with the sailors.

" 'The one I love,' she says, 'is a sailor of the earth. And every day he discovers new isles. He will bring them to us in his hand, warm and singing like nests of birds. You will see. He is not wicked: he tries but he does not know how to be.'

"She squeezes my hand; her thoughts have gone far into the wide world.

" 'He must still be alive,' she says. 'I marked my thickly rouged lips on a piece of paper and he must have kept it. It was his passport to hope.'

"Then she takes five glasses from the sideboard. She arranges them on the tray. She opens her perfume box and in it there is a new jar, and at once I smell an odor. She has not taken the lid off yet, but I know that the seeds are in it, in that iron-colored paste that lies heavy in the bottom.

"She makes a lemonade with fine fresh lemons. She had someone buy her some ice and that was very expensive in our hot country, but she had sold her necklace that smelled like the stone quarry. With her spatula she puts in the bottom of each glass a tiny kernel of the iron-colored paste. She pours in the lemon juice and spring water. She puts in a little shaving of ice, then she says, 'Come, let's look at the boats. Let's forget the world!'

"It was necessary to climb up on the cupboard. We

reached the high window and we saw the port. It was the first time I had seen it but my mother knew it well.

"Our palace rose sheer from the water like a rock and the sailboats would come and be moored to our wall. There was a lovely pure white three-master, the *Adelaide*. Her long slack cable floated in the water. From time to time the boat would give a great tug at the cable and the cable would smoke in the sun like a spurt of fire. But our palace did not budge. A small boat groaned as it pressed forward with its poop. Looking at our wall all plastered with seaweed eyebrows down below, it seemed to me that our house was a face grounded in the sea, that the vessels attached to its forehead were going to pull all together to draw it out of the water and that at last, the mouth would emerge to tell our misfortune to the world.

"The *Adelaide* was indeed doing her best; the little boat also. Only one little ship called the *Ouraba* was doing nothing. The Aztec who equipped it used it to fish for devilfish.

"My mother sang to herself a wild song that she invented as she went along:

The brow of my love is harnessed to the sailboats.
My love is a real man. I did not know that he was
   real, but now, I know, I know.
My beloved is full of children and I did not want
   them and I was wrong, and now I know that I
   want them.

"Then she jumped down off the cupboard and gave me her hand, saying, 'Come, it is ready.'

"She took the tray in her hands and went toward the old people's room.

"The odor of the seeds cried aloud in the palace. So loudly that Angiolina put her hands over her ears.

"When my mother entered the room, Monseigneur began to laugh.

"'I have brought you something to drink,' said my mother.

"'Who opened the door?' said Madame Horatius.

"'Oh, Simiane, to us who love you so!' sighed Madame Captain.

"My mother stood there trembling before them.

"'We must punish her,' said Monsieur Horatius.

"'And severely,' added Monsieur Captain, 'for it is poison. Punish her, Monseigneur, you have the right.'

"My father took a glass from the tray and he held it out to my mother.

"'Drink,' he said.

"And she drank, but she did not look at me."

After a silence, Odripano added, "Besides, the one who lived on the hill of Fiesole was already dead and they had buried him with his passport of hope."

This time it was indeed the escape. My body was still there, in the town: it was the part that had left the *collège* and was kept now in a bank. It was made to sit at a table, it copied addresses. They gave it letters, it delivered them. They called to it: "Go, open the door for Madame."

And I went and opened the door for Madame and Madame passed out without having to trouble to touch the door, so she could with no inconvenience look at the gold pieces in her hands, rubbing them gently between her thumb and her forefinger before putting them into her purse. She could do all that: I held the door. I had a fine light blue suit. Yes, in spite of everything, the distributor of chance had chosen for me the Comptoir d'Escompte where the livery was blue. There are laws which even chance is forced to follow.

I said with a bow, "Good day, Madame."

She did not look at me. The director looked at me to see if the angle of the body was sufficiently deferential. He called to me: "Come here. You must bend over a little more. Not too much, but just a little more: dignified politeness. Like this."

And he did it. Very good!

"Do you understand?"

Yes, I understood. I had divided myself into two parts, each with all the wheels. There were twenty or thirty little wheels in my head to which I had given the task of understanding dignified politeness and beautiful penmanship. All that part of the mechanism was called "Come here" and it earned thirty francs a month, and that bought the potatoes.

The greater part nothing could touch. It was called "Blue Boy." They would have loved to catch it and shut it up in the livery that bowed to the ladies. But it was too late. Already the face on the wall, Décidément and Madame-la-Reine, Anne and the girl perfumed with musk, all those had one after the other helped it escape to fair pastures.

Franchesc Odripano had given it spurs of swallow wings, and now it was astride the steed.

I lived in a bitter and exalted world. It seems that all the princesses had been rescued without waiting for me. It was the time of my flowering. I had need of heroism, love, and bruising. At my every gesture the gift of myself flowed through my veins like sweat.

However, I would sometimes go to my father's work-room where he was deep in thought. He had stopped the work he was holding in his hands.

"What are you thinking about?"

He would look at me with his velvet eyes.

"Of the kings who used to heal the 'king's evil.' "

"What about them?"

"Well, son, they healed the 'king's evil.' That is all, and to do it they had only to touch the evil with their finger. Sometimes they could make a leper clean. They had only to pass their hand over the sore, caress the leper as one does a cat, rubbing the fur the wrong way, and the scales would fall and the flesh lose its swelling."

He spoke softly through his beard.

"To heal! To comfort!"

Then: "A man," he said, "who had that power and who wasted his time in anything else: in rendering justice, for instance! That is an excuse for revolutions!

"When a person has a pure breath," my father said, "he can put out wounds all about him like so many lamps."

But I was not so sure. I said, "If you put out all the lamps, Papa, you won't be able to see any more."

At that moment the velvet eyes were still and they were looking beyond my glorious youth.

"That is true," he replied, "the wounds illumine. That is true. You listen to Odripano a good deal. He has had experience. If he can stay young amongst us it is because he is a poet. Do you know what poetry is? Do you know that what he says is poetry? Do you know that, son? It is essential to realize that. Now listen. I, too, have had my experiences, and I tell you that you must put out the wounds. If, when you get to be a man, you know these two things, poetry and the science of extinguishing wounds, then you *will* be a man."

I did not know that everything he was saying then was going on ahead of me along my way to wait for me, and I was thinking of Franchesc, of his forehead that the sailboats had pulled from the sea.

Summer had come again and it was necessary to rest after the noonday meal. The town was all burned and dry. There was no water in the fountains. Along the walls the plaster cracked and fell in great scales. The dust was alive in the streets; a thick layer of powdered earth stirred beneath our feet. Sometimes a heavy breath flowed down from the mountains and the whole town smoked like a cloud of fire. The men all had white moustaches and the women's eyebrows were no longer visible. The houses rotted beneath it and a golden pus oozed from the sinks. In the district where the garbage was dumped, typhoid fever had sown its seeds and nearly every house had a victim wrapped in its cocoon of sheets and blankets, shriveled

and shivering. They no longer rang the bells for the dead.
When the sun set behind the hills, a vast pale light still
hung for some time in the sky and the men set out to seek
water in the hills. When they returned they would stop at
the edge of town in the first olive groves and rest beneath
the stars. They could not roll cigarettes for the tobacco had
all gone to powder. They smoked white clay pipes.

Odripano went to sleep immediately after lunch. He left
his door open.

I go in. He is lying on his big leather mattress. He is tall
and thin. He is lying on his back. He has no stomach. At
the place where all men of his age have rolls of fat, I see
under his shirt that the skin is hollow. He has linen trousers
on. His feet are bare. His chest is broad with two strong
breast muscles, and between them is a great ravine where
the muscles are attached in a mysterious thick shrubbery of
gray hair. He is breathing slowly, deeply, silently. He takes
a deep breath as if he were about to wake up, then he gradually lets it out again. He has no pillow under his head and
the skin of his neck is smooth. He had shaved this morning.
His chin is nothing but skin and bones. It might have been
rather plump in its youth. Now it is dried up and like the
prow of a boat. The yellow skin clings tightly to the bone,
but at the point there is still a little dimple, like a thumb
mark in plaster. The mouth is narrow. The upper lip, thin
as a thread, curves and points in the middle; it turns down
at the edges around the lower lips, swells again, a little dried
by age, but it must have been fleshy and thick, and secret.
It has nothing left to hide. One feels that it has been joyless
for a long time. There is no color left in that gray mouth,

and now in sleep, no strength. It is making a grimace. Franchesc has two profiles. If I look at him from the right, his regular nose, curved in an eagle beak, gives roundness and nobility to that triangular face. From the left, the nose inclines over the cheek. Sensuality, cunning yet full of tenderness, is hidden in the shadow of that nose. On that side the face has a great power of love and suffering; on that side Franchesc Odripano resembles Francis the First. His eyes are closed. He has no cheeks. There, too, the skin is tight over the bones. The death mask has long been rising in the soul and the flesh and it is on the level with the skin. It no longer waits for a signal to emerge with its vines, its tigers, and its mounts of serpents. The eyes are closed. Franchesc will not be very changed in death from the way he looks now, here before me. He simply will not breathe any more, and that will not make a great difference, for I listen in vain, I cannot hear his breath, I see only his breast slowly rising and falling. He has finished his life; his other-world face is already formed. His eyes are closed. The mouth will disappear, that is all. And not even the whole mouth; that upper lip will harden and remain; it is the lower lip that will crumble because it will no longer be able to taste the sweetness of the earth. It knows it. It is already prepared. But, in spite of the closed eyes—and even sleep cannot prevent the flicker of the eyelids like featherless birds—a gleam filters between the lashes.

He told me that once in Rome he fell asleep on a couch. He was visiting. They had said, "Lie down." He had lain down and fallen asleep immediately, as usual: like a diver, he said. It was in the house of the woman he loved. "She went off, I believe, to finish her toilet and her friend stayed beside me to watch me. I was, it seems, as still as death and I breathed so lightly that that friend became alarmed. Then, when she sensed the rhythm of my breathing with its depth and peacefulness, she discovered that she, too, felt a deep peace. She clasped her hands on her knees, sat back in the armchair and stayed there watching over me. Between us was a little low stand and on this stand a lighted candle, for the woman I loved had taken away the lamp."

When Franchesc told a story, he always designated the characters by some sensual trait they had in relation to him and he would repeat this designation throughout the tale. "It is revealing," he would say. Now, he repeated: "For the woman I loved had taken away the lamp.

"Then, while we were alone, I raised my arm. That was done, it seems, without a start or any emotion, just the arm, heavily, slowly. A gesture from outside. A gesture that did not have its place traced in advance in the air that evening. And then I let it fall squarely on the candle. The woman who was watching me did not stir, and after a moment the woman I loved returned. And she said, 'What are you two doing? Why isn't there any light here?'

"I heard someone saying, 'He did it. He put the light out with a blow of his fist.'

"Then I awoke and the rest doesn't matter."

Franchesc is sleeping. His arms lying close to his sides do not move. I look at this room so clean and bare. He had filled up all the nail holes in the walls before whitewashing them. There is about him neither flaw nor weakness. The deal table, the two chairs, that leather cushion like those on

which a veterinarian lays horses for gelding. That is all.
A faint suggestion of scrolls on the leather cushion that
serves as the man's bed. All around that, outside, the town
both baked and rotting, the town that smells like a piece of
spoiled meat that has been put to grill on the coals, the town
with its typhoid patients, its manure heaps, and the splendid
woolen covering of pink and gray roofs.

Franchesc does not move. I wait. Perhaps he will lift an
arm, heavily, slowly, in one of those unexpected gestures.
Perhaps the one who is behind him, who knows the past
and the future, and who sees all of life from top to bottom
like the wheel of a rainbow on the sea, perhaps that one
will make him make another of those unworldly gestures
fraught with meaning. I wait. He does not stir. He has
finished. There is nothing left to explain to him. It is not
worth the trouble. There remains nothing for him but sleep.
Nothing more.

I look at you, Franchesc, I look at that dead face that is
slowly rising through the flesh. It is already there under the
transparent skin, with its bones. The light of your forehead
is growing dim; your white woolly hair is lying like ripe
grain, your dingy skin is exuding the brownish sweat of age.
In you there is no longer a man, there is only the material
for a hundred new grasshoppers, ten lizards, three snakes,
a fine patch of lush grass, and perhaps the heart of a tree.
I bend over you as over the reflection in a mirror.

I made the acquaintance of love and friendship almost at
the same time. My mother's employes were now of my age.
The two Louisas had already gone. Antonine could be seen

from time to time going wearily down the street. Three
other girls had come to take their places. You cannot put
hens and roosters together without making eggs. Marie-
Jeanne and I learned about love together. Sunday afternoon I would go and wait for her in a road on the hill between two high banks. She would come. I could hear her
step a long way off. Finally she would emerge from the
trees. I remember she wore a red flannel blouse with white
dots. I knew a little grotto encircled by the branches of an
old fig tree. There the ground was covered with fine sand.
There was nothing to soil one; nothing. We kissed each
other a long time and then I touched her. It was an enormous new happiness to feel her skin beneath my hand, her
sensitive breasts, her little ankle, her calves, her thighs, that
fruit of warm animal life. Then she lay down.

Franchesc Odripano gave me a poem.

I met my father on the stairs. He had a newspaper in his
hand.

"Have you seen?" he said. "Have you seen? The American has flown!"

"What do you mean, flown?"

"In the air."

He spread his arms and began to wave them like wings.
"Fifty meters," he said.

Downstairs, the wife of the pork butcher had bought a
new machine. It was wound with a key. You put a wax
cylinder on it and it played "You Who Know the Hussars
of the Guard." She was down there playing it.

"You hear," he said to me, "that, and then to fly like the

birds, and then the magic lantern. . . . Just wait, you are young, you will see."

We were on the landing. Odripano came to his door.

"What is it, Père Jean?"

My father held out the newspaper.

"The American has flown."

"Ah! yes," he said.

"Doesn't that interest you?"

"No, not at all."

"But it's something, all the same."

"No," said Odripano, "it isn't anything. Let's get it straight. It isn't anything because it will change nothing."

"What!" said my father. "It won't change anything? Just consider. I'm not saying that fifty meters is the end of the world, nor of the event either, but it is enormous for today. Tomorrow it will be fifty kilometers, then, who knows—"

"*I*, I know," said Odripano.

"What do you know?"

"I know that it will surely be fifty kilometers, and perhaps even five hundred or five thousand kilometers—"

"Oh! Five *thousand*," said my father.

"Yes, five thousand, fifty thousand if you like. They can go to the moon; it won't change anything."

"Do you think so?" said my father. "Why?"

"Because the whole happiness of man is in the little valleys."

Against the wall beside us was a swallow's nest and the mothers were coming to feed their babies.

"Yes," said Odripano. "Let's sit down on the stairs, Père Jean, you have a moment. There is one thing that is the great tragedy of life."

"Sit down, son," said my father.

"Yes, of life. It is that we are only in halves. From the time we began to build houses and cities, since we invented the wheel, we have not advanced one step toward happiness. We have always been in halves. As long as we invent and progress in mechanical things and not in love, we shall not achieve happiness."

"Go on," said my father, "I am listening." And he filled his pipe.

"You understand, I care nothing about your flying machine if half my heart is bleeding because it lacks the other half, the one without which it will never be one of the fine fruits of the earth. Do you see what I mean?"

"I see."

"All those magic carpets, they will bring cargoes of sorrows and terrible things, as long as you expect sensitivity and love of them. Don't let this boy have too much hope, unless you are training him for a business career."

My father began to laugh. "Yes, I am training him for business, all business, in the plural."

Odripano gently patted my father's knee with the palm of his hand.

"Cobbler after my own heart," he said. "I know that you are as strong as I in that. Not stronger, but as strong. That is why you disturbed me just now with your newspaper.

"You know where things ought to be invented? In the

call, in the voice, in the sound that comes from the heart. I have been in the Tyrol and in the Aosta valley. Every time there is a moon the deer come out of the forest. They stand at the grassy edge, they lift their heads and they call. From my bedroom I could see them, all white in the distance. Once I had gone from the village of Santoretto and as I was passing through the woods I also heard the roe calling softly. I have lived in Fiesole, on the hill. Do you know a lizard's voice? It sounds like when you run your nail over the ribs of corduroy trousers. And the mole crickets at night? And the birds, and all? Everything seeks its like, everything calls to its own.

"The great curse of heaven upon us has been to make our hearts each one different from the other. One for each one of us. Once divided in two, it is necessary to find your identical half. Without it you are alone all your life long. That is the tragedy. You cannot imagine the number of those whose hearts are incomplete.

"You want me to predict what will happen, and the boy will see it if he lives. Well, listen. At the great moment of hope, magic is going bankrupt. Your flying carpets will be loaded with potatoes and carrots. People will say to themselves: 'What! We are not happier?' You are not happier because you have invented nothing new in the call that you make around you in your search for the other half of your heart. You still make your small voice of the cave age. Much smaller. And you will not find it. Then people will kill their hearts because it will be too difficult to live with them.

"You see, cobbler, bad news in your newspaper."

"Well," said my father, "perhaps there are some left who will keep on calling, eh, son?"

"Yes," said Odripano, "*I* am still calling. Nevertheless I know that I shall no longer be heard."

"And now that we have settled the question, to work," said my father. "You have made a fine speech about the heart but said little about the stomach."

I was standing alone on the stairs watching the swallows when Odripano called me softly from his room.

"Come here, lad."

He had opened the drawer of his deal table and had taken out a big copybook that had no cover. On the first page he had written "Franchesc Odripano," and then "*I sposi*." He handed me a sheet of paper.

"Here," he said, "I have copied this for you and I have translated it because it is in Italian. I understand better what I say in my own tongue.

"It is to continue what we were talking about," he said. "Remember, all of man's happiness is in the little valleys. Tiny little ones. Small enough to call from one side to the other."

I looked at the sheet. It was a poem by Saint Francis to Saint Claire:

Do you hear the bell, Saint Claire?
I had stuffed it with grass and dirt so that the clapper would stop striking and I slept on my folded arm to annul my strength. And now I would call you, and I strike the bronze with the bone of my fist so that my voice may fly beyond the hills.
Do you hear the bell, Saint Claire?

No, for they have cut off your ears and stuffed the holes with honey as they do with fighting cranes to make them fierce and bellicose.

> Franchesc Odripano
> —I sposi.

I don't remember how my friendship for Louis David began. At this moment as I speak of him, I can no longer recall my pure youth, the enchantment of the magicians and of the days. I am steeped in blood. Beyond this book there is a deep wound from which all men of my age are suffering. This side of the page is soiled with pus and darkness.

He left shortly before me in August 1914. His father and I accompanied him to the station. Beyond a thicket of trees the engine was puffing. He said to me, "You go back now. Don't come all the way. I don't want to see you when we pull out."

And I kissed him there on the road.

In July 1916 I returned from Verdun with hospital leave. My mother was waiting for me at the station. There was no more "Golden Wheat" and "Griefs Are Mad Things." Her poor blond hair was ashy gray. We went up toward the town through the meadows. It was beautiful weather. There were bees everywhere. I asked, "And Papa? And everybody?"

She stopped and said to me, "Paul Hode was killed."

And after several more steps: "Be brave. David is dead!"

Be brave!

I have here before me that memorandum book that he left me. I know that in the little pocket of the cover there is a lock of woman's hair. I have just looked at it. It is falling to pieces.

I open the book! "Memorandum for the year 1913."

January first, Wednesday, Circumcision:
   Trajectory is the curve described by the ball in its flight through space.
   Line of fire is the axis of the barrel indefinitely prolonged.
   Objective is the. . . .

He wrote that!
They made him write that!

My poor Louis! Life is all about this little room where I am writing. Listen to the poplar and the south wind. Smell that odor of oak logs. Look! Outside the window the whole dark plain is alight. It is night. The farms down there are burning dry leaves, carts are rumbling along the roads. A timid girl is singing beneath the willows as she feels about in the dark to gather in the washing. I know that you are there, behind me, always. Behind me now as I write. I know that your friendship is more faithful than all the loves in the world and that it is, humbly, of another quality. But I want you to have your place among all those who can pick apples, eat figs, run, swim, beget urchins, live.

More selfishly, Louis, I want you here for my own sake. I listen. There is not a sound here. Only outside, the rain and the wind are beginning. Here, here, where are you? Over there in the shadow of the bureau there is only my bed. That dark object yonder is my shepherd's cape. I'll go and see. No, nothing but my cape and my scarf and my beret. Empty, my beret. No skull inside: soft. You are not here. Where are you then? In front of my books, those two or three that you would always pick up and stand reading? Are you there? I touch the books. The dust is still on them. Louis, I tell you, I need you this evening. This evening, and every day that has passed without you, and every day to come, I need your friendship. Oh! I *have* looked, old man. Do you remember the time we used to talk about all those things up in the hills? I have sought like that. You know what I must have offered. You saw me? You know what they did with it. No, I need you. And where can I look for you? I feel your presence in my heart, but I know that I would have peace if I could see you here in the armchair smoking your pipe.

If you had only died for honorable things; if you had fought for love or in getting food for your little ones. But, no. First they deceived you and then they killed you in the war.

What do you want me to do with this France that you have helped, it seems, to preserve, as I, too, have done? What shall we do with it, we who have lost all our friends? Ah! If it were a question of defending rivers, hills, mountains, skies, winds, rains, I would say, "Willingly. That is our job. Let us fight. All our happiness in life is there." No, we have defended the sham name of all that. When I see a river, I say 'river'; when I see a tree, I say 'tree'; I never say 'France.' That does not exist.

Ah! How willingly would I give away that false name that one single one of those dead, the simplest, the most humble, might live again! Nothing can be put into the scales with the human heart. They are all the time talking about God! It is God who gave the tiny shove with His finger to the pendulum of the clock of blood at the instant the child dropped from its mother's womb. They are always talking about God, when the only product of His good workmanship, the only thing that is godlike, the life that He alone can create, in spite of all your science of bespectacled idiots, that life you destroy at will in an infamous mortar of slime and spit, with the blessing of all your churches. What logic.

There is no glory in being French. There is only one glory: in being alive.

You are a shadow there, behind my chair. I shall never touch your hand again. You will never lean against my shoulder. I shall never hear your voice again; never see your good face with its honesty and its broad smile. I know that you are there, near me, as are all the dead I have loved and who have loved me, like my father, like one or two others.

But you are dead.

I do not hate the one who killed you with a bullet through your stomach. They deceived him as they deceived you. They told him that the rivers were named 'Germany.' They made him write in his note book: "Objective is the. . . ."

I hate the one who dictated.

I had two more long conversations with my father. He was ill. A sort of somber, dull pain was eating his liver. He did not complain. We only felt that he was sorely stricken in the softest, the most vital part of his being. He had grown thin. His beard filled his face out a little, but when he came back from the barber's, he entered with a strange face that grew more and more bony. His hand, as it left the doorknob, floated a moment, imponderable, in the air. His eyes looked through things and he took several soft swaying steps as if he were walking on a cloud.

"What are you looking at me for?"

My mother tried to speak with her trembling lips: "Just to see you, Père, that's all."

"Do I please you?"

He had become cruel and hard. His thin mouth was gnawed by a kind of acrid fever and was nothing but a trickle of vinegar under his moustache.

For some years past we had a little garden on the hillside. The land and the olive trees had cost a hundred and fifty francs. My father had had a brick hut built and a well dug beneath a linden, a chestnut, and a cypress. He went out there every day. He fed his rabbits. Sometimes I would go furtively. I would hide behind the honeysuckle. It was then that my father developed the habit of humming with his mouth closed, a dull sound, devoid of form or color, monotonous, restrained, strangely magnetic, that was as haunting as the beat of a distant drum.

We were sitting under the linden tree. He put his hand on my arm.

"Son," he said, "I must talk to you a little. I have been wanting to for some time. I think a lot. I am alone. I think of many things. I will not be here when you are a man. No, you are not a man yet. One learns little by little. We have gone along together until now."

He sat silent a moment, humming.

"It is not hard to live alone, son. The hard thing is to suffer alone. That is why so many seek God. When they have found Him, they are no longer alone. Only, listen to me, they do not find Him, they invent Him.

"What one wants in one's heart, even when one is suffering acutely, is to continue. To live. Even when one dies, one wants to keep on existing. Yes, living: to keep on living. Another life. The life beyond, paradise, no matter what you call it. Yes, at the place where the road enters the shadow, we put a mirror. Instead of looking at what there is beyond, of accustoming ourselves to the shadow, we set up a mirror. In this glass it is this side of life that we see: the road we have just come over and which seems to be going on through the mirror. It is slightly blurred, slightly mysterious, a little faint, as are all reflections. It imitates the beyond very well. There are trees, sky, earth, clouds, wind, life. Life. That is what we want.

"That is all very well as long as one is on this side of the mirror. But as soon as one goes beyond—you see, a glass is not very thick, no thicker than my finger—well, as soon as one takes a step on the other side, then suddenly one knows. One knows that it is lies, deception; one cries out. . . . Sometimes people say: 'His death was terribly hard.' What is there on the other side? I don't know. I might say, nothing. I do not believe that there is nothing. I do not know. I won't tell you there isn't anything. The moment one knows, one utters a cry, and there you are. That is not the point.

"When one succeeds in inventing God, here is the God one invents. He is beside you. He watches over you, caresses you. You are the most beautiful. It seems that you are the only one in the world. He is your father and your mother. When you do wrong, He corrects you. When you do right, He puts some candies in a box and says to you: 'This is for you later on.' He is like the man who walks before the oxen with a handful of salt to make them go forward in the plowing when it is difficult and who leads them to the slaughter house with the same handful of salt. They have invented a God like that. He promises you everything, my son, the mirror promises, too.

"Only, the time that you spend beside your invention, everything is pleasant. I admit it is agreeable to be able to talk to someone, to complain, to ask, to groan. And I don't know whether in the long run it is not better to invent God, to shut one's eyes and ears, to say a thousand times over: 'It is true, it is true, He exists.' And then to believe it. I do not know.

"Because, son, the terrible thing is to suffer alone. You will discover that later."

He filled his pipe.

"Where I made a mistake, was when I wanted to be good and helpful. You will make a mistake, like me."

He began to puff gently on his pipe and to hum that monotonous tune that enveloped him like the silk of a cocoon.

Blue Boy

He talked to me a second time in the presence of a wonderful sunset. It was like a vast harvest stirred by the wind. Sheaves of clouds piled high in the hollows of the hills. An impalpable golden grain waved over the celestial stalks. The sun with its rays was rooted in the mud like a broken wheel.

"Once," said my father—that day he was very calm, very handsome, with his poor face of gray clay deeply hollowed by death—"once I subscribed to an illustrated magazine. It was very interesting. It had a little of everything in it. There was reading matter: 'The Arm of Steel,' 'The Mysteries of Paris,' 'The Wandering Jew.' On the two middle pages there were reproductions of paintings, statues. I used to cut them out to put in my workroom. The Venus de Milo, and then a big sort of fellow stiff and straight like a tree trunk, a victor in a chariot race. It was in that magazine that one day I found a beautiful picture. First, in the foreground, there was a gigantic man. You could see his bare leg. His calves were bound by muscles as thick as my thumb. In one hand he was holding a scythe and in the other some sprays of wheat. He was looking at the wheat. Just by looking at his mouth you could tell that in harvesting the wheat he killed partridges. You were sure that he loved plump roast partridges and heavy blue wine, the kind that leaves a cloud in the glass and in the mouth. Behind him—you see, it is rather hard to explain—behind him, imagine a great landscape like this, bigger than this because the artist put everything in, he had mingled everything to show that what he wanted to paint was the whole world. A river, a river that flowed through forests, mead-

ows, fields, cities, villages. A river that finally fell in the distance in a great cascade. On the river, boats sailed from
one bank to the other, barges slept, and the water was
covered with little wrinkles about them, rafts of logs
floated down the current. On the bridges men were fishing.
In the villages the chimneys were smoking, bells were ringing, showing their noses in the belfries. In the cities there
was a teeming of vehicles. From one port on the river great
boats were sailing away. Some were at rest in a little bay
in the meadow, others hesitating at the edge of the river
current, still others already swept along by this force toward the sea. On the shore there was calm, just ruffled
enough to show the foam breaking over some vast fish cast
up on the sand. Some men were cutting up these fish with
picks, others were carrying great strips of flesh on their
shoulders toward their homes. The housewives were standing at their doors watching them. In the houses the hearth
fires were burning. One young girl was putting her little
brother to bed. In another window you could see a youth
urging a girl toward a bed. In the forests men were cutting
down trees. In the farms they were killing the pig. Children
were dancing about a drunkard. An old woman was crying out her window that someone was stealing her chickens.
A midwife came out of a house to wash her hands at the
brook. An old hag was asking her to return her scissors.
The father was smoking his pipe. The young mother had
her head turned away so as not to see what was going on.
Blankets were warming before the hearth. On another fire
they were cooking meat. On another corpses were being
burned. The fields were teeming with work. Men were

plowing, others sowing, harvesting, gathering in the grapes, threshing the grain, winnowing, kneading the dough, dragging the oxen forward, beating the donkey, reining in the horse, raising the hoe, the ax, the pick, or pressing so hard against the plow that their sabots dropped in the furrow.

"All that!

"It interested me enormously. It was called 'The Fall of Icarus.'

"At first I said to myself: 'They've put the wrong title.' I looked for a while and then I got to work at my shoemaking.

"All day long, son, all day long, I said to myself: 'The Fall of Icarus, the Fall of Icarus! Icarus who slew a thousand cocks and a thousand hens, eagles, and other birds, and who glued the feathers on his arms, the down on his breast, and then tried to fly. Where is he? They have the wrong title!'

"No.

"That evening I lit my lamp and I looked. It was all right.

"High up in the middle of the sky, above all that teeming life, that was not looking, that was unknowing, all that was living life to its full, high above it all, Icarus was falling.

"He was as big as this, look, as the tip of my fingernail. Black, one arm here, a leg there, lost, like a little dead monkey.

"He was falling."

My father's thin hand made a gesture to indicate that it had no importance.

After a moment he added, "Remember that, my son."

We entered the year '14 without being aware of it. It gently went its round of snows, swallows, blossoming almond trees. The wheat grew as usual. The wild tulips appeared on time; they came peacefully out of the old bulbs of the spring of '13. The swallows found their old nests. The hares had troops of baby rabbits. The barriers were enlarged around the sheepfolds, because that year the seed of the rams had been well sown; there were almost a third more lambs. The grass grew much better than the preceding year and more lush. The creatures pastured in it took a joy in eating. They chewed a long time, looking up at the sky. The earth was easy to cultivate. It had rained just enough. The wind had been right. All was peace. Peace and joy rose from the heart of the earth through the grass, through the trees, through the long veins of the hares, the foxes, the wild boars, the rams, the ewes, and the males sowed peaceful, living seed like the Milky Way. The wheel of the world turned noiselessly in its thick oil.

The men were restless. Things were too good. It left them a great deal of time for their men's cares. The earth spurted so richly, like a fine well-nourished breast, that one drank without thinking of caressing it and drawing one's pleasure from that. One considered nothing but mental agility, and in each clan they looked every morning voluptuously at the old men, those skilful in speech, clever in ruling, cunning in hiding their thirst for wealth and whose heads were inflated like soap bubbles. Each clan took pride in having the biggest bubbles. The poets went no more to the fields, they slobbered in their trumpets. During this time, the earth's milk was streaming through all growing things and the glory of the beasts and the trees increased. The men, too well-fed, had forgotten their powers of procreation; they were uniting with gasoline, phosphates, things without thighs. This gave them a thirst for blood.

It was easy for me to set out for the war without any great feeling of emotion, simply because I was young, and over all young men they were blowing a wind that sang of pirates and the ocean sail.